Authoring Patient Records
An Interactive Guide

Michael P. Pagano, PA-C, PhD
Assistant Professor
Director, Graduate Program
Department of Communication
Fairfield University
Fairfield, Connecticut

Chapter 7 by
Canera L. Pagano, RN, JD
Associate
Wilson Elser Moskowitz Edelman & Dicker, LLP
Stamford, Connecticut

JONES AND BARTLETT PUBLISHERS
Sudbury, Massachusetts
BOSTON   TORONTO   LONDON   SINGAPORE

World Headquarters

Jones and Bartlett Publishers	Jones and Bartlett Publishers	Jones and Bartlett Publishers
40 Tall Pine Drive	Canada	International
Sudbury, MA 01776	6339 Ormindale Way	Barb House, Barb Mews
978-443-5000	Mississauga, Ontario L5V 1J2	London W6 7PA
info@jbpub.com	Canada	United Kingdom
www.jbpub.com		

Jones and Bartlett's books and products are available through most bookstores and online book-sellers. To contact Jones and Bartlett Publishers directly, call 800-832-0034, fax 978-443-8000, or visit our website, www.jbpub.com.

Substantial discounts on bulk quantities of Jones and Bartlett's publications are available to corporations, professional associations, and other qualified organizations. For details and specific discount information, contact the special sales department at Jones and Bartlett via the above contact information or send an email to specialsales@jbpub.com.

This publication is designed to provide accurate and authoritative information in regard to the Subject Matter covered. It is sold with the understanding that the publisher is not engaged in rendering legal, accounting, or other professional service. If legal advice or other expert assistance is required, the service of a competent professional person should be sought.

Production Credits

Publisher: David Cella
Associate Editor: Maro Gartside
Editorial Assistant: Teresa Reilly
Production Manager: Julie Champagne Bolduc
Associate Production Editor:
  Jessica Steele Newfell
Marketing Manager: Grace Richards

Manufacturing and Inventory Control
  Supervisor: Amy Bacus
Composition: Glyph International
Cover Design: Kristin E. Parker
Cover Image: © 3DProfi/ShutterStock, Inc.
Printing and Binding: Malloy, Inc.
Cover Printing: Malloy, Inc.

Library of Congress Cataloging-in-Publication Data
Pagano, Michael P.
  Authoring patient records : an interactive guide / Michael P. Pagano ;
with contributions by Canera L. Pagano.
     p. ; cm.
  Includes bibliographical references and index.
  ISBN 978-0-7637-6321-3 (pbk. : alk. paper)
  1. Medical records. 2. Medical history taking. I. Pagano, Canera L. II. Title.
  [DNLM: 1. Medical Records—Problems and Exercises. 2.
Communication—Problems and Exercises. 3. Documentation—methods—Problems
and Exercises. 4. Medical History Taking—methods—Problems and Exercises.
WX 18.2 P131a 2011]
  R864.P355 2011
  610—dc22

                                             2010001247

6048

Printed in the United States of America
14 13 12 11 10   10 9 8 7 6 5 4 3 2 1

To my sons, Brian and Anthony, for giving my life a purpose. —Michael

To my mother, Jené, for inspiring me to become a nurse and to my Grandpa Oren, whose tales of being a judge and a lawyer motivated me to follow in his footsteps. —Canera

Contents

Preface

The purpose of *Authoring Patient Records: An Interactive Guide* is to help healthcare providers—medical doctors, doctors of osteopathy, physician assistants, advanced practice registered nurses, physical therapists—learn and practice a process for authoring patient records. In addition, this book is intended to be used by health communication researchers, students, and scholars in their evaluations of written or electronic communication about patients' illnesses, injuries, treatments, prognoses, and interactions with healthcare providers.

It should be noted that this text is not intended to replace current texts and pedagogy related to the content required in specific medical records for various healthcare professionals. Therefore, this book assumes that readers will have a fundamental understanding of the medical terms and clinical skills required to interview and care for patients as well as the knowledge of what information about the patient interaction and clinical findings need to be documented in a specific patient record. The focus of this book is on helping providers enhance their communication effectiveness, credibility, and professionalism as well as minimize their malpractice risks.

The goal of this text is to make the writing process—whether on paper, dictated, or computerized—clear, concise, and effective. The author, a physician assistant (PA), has a 30-year history of creating, reading, and researching written, computerized, and dictated patient records. His PA experience includes working in surgery, primary care, women's health, emergency departments, and occupational medicine. In addition, the author has taught writing and health communication courses in universities and professional programs for more than two decades. He has published three books and numerous journal articles related to healthcare writing and communication.

This book is designed to be a truly interactive text. It can be used by an individual, in a course, or in a small group setting. Throughout the text, you will find boxes to help you assess your understanding of the topics covered in the chapter as well as blank spaces and exercises for you to practice the authoring process being discussed. The answers to these questions can be found in the text that follows them, so try to answer the questions first and then compare your responses to the material in the text. It is important for you to recognize that authoring (whether with pen, pencil, dictation, or computer) is a skill, and, like all skills, it requires assimilation, organization, critical analysis, and practice. It is frequently argued by healthcare providers that modern medical constraints (healthcare maintenance organizations, workload, and institutional policies) limit their time for patient interaction and documentation. This text will offer tips for enhancing your record, keeping with minimal time extensions, but it will also demonstrate and illustrate the importance of effective documentation for quality care, safety, continuity of care, and legal reasons.

In addition, this book includes a unique chapter dedicated to improving your knowledge about malpractice risks related to medical record authorship. Chapter 7 was authored by a registered nurse (RN) with two decades of experience working in community hospitals, emergency medicine, and postanesthesia recovery units. Furthermore, the RN/JD author has more than 5 years of experience as a medical malpractice defense attorney. This chapter includes discussions of how authors can create patient records that provide the information needed by users of the documents without increasing the provider's legal risks.

NOTE: The examples of patient records used in this text are anonymous, real documents obtained from a wide variety of healthcare institutions nationwide.

Reviewer Recognition

Nancy D. Allen, CCC-SLP
Communication Disorders and Sciences Department
State University of New York at Plattsburgh

Linda Biggers, PT, CLT
Director of PTA Program
Krannert School of Physical Therapy
University of Indianapolis

Melissa J. Coffman, MPA, PA-C
Physician Assistant Department Chair
Nova Southeastern University, Fort Lauderdale

Daniel Curtis, PT, MS
Program Director
PTA Program
Arkansas Tech University–Ozark Campus

Lora L. Davis, PT, MS, DPT
Department of Physical Therapy
Arizona School of Health Sciences
A.T. Still University

Raymond Eifel, MS, PA-C
Assistant Professor
Division of Physician Assistant Studies
Shenandoah University

Tina Patel Gunaldo, PT, DPT, MHS
Clinical Instructor
School of Allied Health Professions
Louisiana State University Health Sciences Center–
    New Orleans

Dawn LaBarbera, PhD, PA-C
Associate Professor
Chair of Department of Physician Assistant Studies
University of Saint Francis

Sharon Dezzani Martin, RN, MSN, CNS-BC, PhD(c)
Associate Professor of Nursing
Department of Nursing
Saint Joseph's College

Judy Ortiz, PA-C, MHS, MS
Associate Director, Associate Professor
School of Physician Assistant Studies
Pacific University

Melissa Patrizi, PT, MS, ATC
Professor
Academic Coordinator of Clinical Education
Remington College–Cleveland West Campus

Michael Pryor, MBA, DC
Director of Clinical Education
Life University

James Scifers, DScPT, PT, SCS, LAT, ATC
Associate Dean
College of Health and Human Sciences
Western Carolina University

Dionne M. Soares, MPAS, PA-C
Physician Assistant Program
College of Pharmacy, Nursing, and Allied Health Sciences
Howard University

Valerie Teglia, PT, DPT, NCS
Director of Clinical Education
Department of Physical Therapy
Mount St. Mary's College

Bridget Tevis, PA-C
Clinical Instructor
Department of Physician Assistant Studies
University of Texas Health Science Center, San Antonio

Jane Trapp, PA-C, MSEd
Clinical Associate Professor
Didactic Education Coordinator
Physician Assistant Program
East Carolina University

Gary R. Uremovich, DMin, MS, MPAS, PA-C
Director
Physician Assistant Program
Wingate University

Chapter 1

The Patient Record: An Overview

It's About Sharing Information

Humans "cannot not communicate" (Watzlawick, Bavelas, & Jackson, 1967, p. 48). This axiom is central to our understanding of the audience's role in all types of communication. Everything humans do, wear, say, don't say, and write communicates to an audience. And, as communication scholars have noted for decades, it does not matter what the sender of a message intended to communicate, only what the audience perceives. The importance of this axiom with respect to this book is that everything a provider–author chooses to include or not include in his or her patient record communicates information not just about the patient's condition or treatment but also about the author. Therefore, understanding the critical role that audiences play in the communication of patient information is central to our work. As you know, professional schools are excellent at teaching future providers the necessary clinical skills to fulfill their particular roles; however, too few of these programs include authoring patient records as a core focus of their educational efforts. This book is intended to help you, either in a classroom, in a team, or individually, to improve your patient record authoring skills and to ensure that you understand what your documents communicate to readers about your patients and your ability and credibility.

Because the patient is the ultimate focus and raison d'être for all healthcare documentation–record keeping, this book will use the term *patient records*, not medical records, throughout. While it may seem an arbitrary, semantic distinction, in fact it is a biopsychosocial determination. Healthcare providers–authors need to consider the documents they create as primarily communicating information about an individual patient—an evolving record of a singular person's health. These documents, like all communication, are a continuous, flexible, history of a person's wellness, illness, or injury that may be used by countless provider and nonprovider readers. By emphasizing a patient-centered focus for these documents, it is the goal of this book to build on the current trend toward patient-centered (as opposed to provider-centered) health communication in all forms (verbal, nonverbal, written, electronic, etc.). In addition, if providers–authors adopt a patient-focused view of the records they create, they are much more likely to communicate more information about the patient, rather than less.

As we begin to discuss authoring patient records, we should understand the history of patient records in the United States. Requirements for maintaining patient records in America can be traced to this country's first hospital. Benjamin Franklin (1754) wrote a book describing the organization and construction of the hospital in Pennsylvania and documented the institution's only requirement for physician's record keeping:

> The practitioner shall keep a fair account (in a book provided for that purpose) of the several patients under their care, of the disorders they labour under, and shall enter in said book the recipes or prescriptions they make for each of them (p. 28).

Initially, the medical record served as a memory device for the patient's physician and as a source of information for other caregivers and the hospital's administrators. For nearly two centuries, these goals and uses for the medical record remained unchanged—it was primarily authored for readers within the author's institution. However, after World War II, the audience, purpose, and use for patient records changed dramatically.

Why would a change in the audience, purpose, and use matter to authors of patient records?

_____

_____

_____

With the postwar baby boom and the increasing shift in population, the patient record began to develop new audiences. These audiences were no longer limited to a single healthcare facility, but instead with the expanding ease of transportation, patients were moving around the country and, therefore, seeking medical care in multiple locales. So, the audience for patient records included future healthcare providers who might practice in cities that were hundreds or even thousands of miles from the record's author. And with this more mobile society, physicians (at the time, the predominant authors and users of patient records) began to demand access to patients' prior records. This change in audience, from only the author to a diverse possibility of readers, necessitated that records be more informative, rather than merely a cryptic memory device for the author.

In addition, with the creation and development of new, larger, and more geographically dispersed hospitals came an even more diverse and expanded audience for patient records. These new facilities brought an astronomic increase in breadth and scope of healthcare providers' roles, including physician assistants, advanced practice nurses, registered nurses, physical therapists, medical technologists, respiratory therapists, among others—all of whom needed access to a patient's health record. As the number of healthcare personnel involved in a patient's care increased, so too did the record's medical and extramedical audiences and the multiple uses for these documents.

> **How does the medical record impact the economics of healthcare delivery?**
>
> _____
>
> _____
>
> _____

As health care continued to develop and expand in the second half of the 20th century, health insurance companies were another audience requiring information about patients. In order for hospitals, clinics, offices, and healthcare providers to receive compensation for their services, insurance companies wanted access to patients' records. This new, extramedical audience created additional concerns for healthcare providers–authors. Suddenly, patient records were not being created to provide information just for other healthcare providers but also for extramedical readers with very different uses for the documents. The need to communicate patient information in a format that could be read and analyzed by insurers might have created too great a burden if the providers–authors did not get reimbursed for their services based on the communication of the medical information.

> **Why are patient records used by malpractice attorneys?**
>
> _____
>
> _____
>
> _____

Contributing further to the growing audiences, purposes, and uses for patient records were the exploding number of medical malpractice lawsuits. As patients complained about their outcomes from healthcare treatment, lawyers, for both the plaintiff (patient or his or her family or estate) and defense (hospital, institution, or provider), became a rapidly expanding new audience for patient records. However, with little or no course work in authoring patient records, healthcare providers frequently found themselves trying to communicate in patient documents not only the information needed by other healthcare providers and insurers but also information that would demonstrate the quality and effectiveness of the care provided for malpractice attorneys.

Furthermore, in the last decade, electronic forms of patient records have evolved and taken a variety of formats. Today, healthcare providers are communicating with and about patients in e-mails, instant messaging, and electronic medical or health records (EMR or EHR). And yet, few providers today are formally trained to author such unique and diverse documents. Nor are these authors educated about the additional risks attributed to creating electronic documents with their ease of dissemination and resulting privacy, regulatory, and legal issues.

The goal of this text is to help providers better understand the importance of the authoring process and how that process can be adapted regardless of the type of healthcare provider or the document or the required audience, purpose, and use. By understanding this process and utilizing it, an author can provide the information needed, in the expected format, and communicate clearly so readers can use the patient records as intended: to inform and persuade readers of the author's thorough evaluation, critical thinking, and credible decision making.

Skills Application

Ask a friend to tell you about his or her weekend or evening. After listening to the narrative, ask any specific questions you need to clarify your understanding of what occurred, where, and why. In the space below, document the story using quotes wherever possible for key elements and work to communicate the information as accurately, concisely, and clearly as possible. Your reader will be a peer (professionally and culturally).

_____

_____

_____

_____

_____

_____

_____

_____

QUESTIONS

1. How did you decide what parts of the story would be important to your reader?

   _____

   _____

2. Did you find it difficult to determine what information to include and what to eliminate in your brief communication? What criteria did you use to make your decisions?

   _____

   _____

   _____

   _____

One of the most difficult tasks for healthcare providers is determining what information a reader needs to understand a patient's problem, the author's analysis, and the treatment plan. The author of patient records needs to meet diverse readers' expectations and still be clear and concise. The following chapters will help you better understand the needs of your audience and what information needs to be communicated to meet the readers' expectations and the document's purpose.

REFERENCES

Franklin, B. (1754). *Some account of the Pennsylvania Hospital: From its first rise to the beginning*. Philadelphia: Franklin & Hall.

Watzlawick, P., Bavelas, J., & Jackson, D. (1967). *Pragmatics of human communication: A study of interactional patterns, pathologies, and paradoxes*. New York, NY: W.W. Norton.

Chapter 2

Audience, Purpose, and Use

Why Document?

In Chapter 1, you documented a story that a friend told you. As you wrote down the information about his or her story, how did you decide what material to include verbatim or in paraphrases or what to leave out? Perhaps you thought about your reader and what he or she might be interested in hearing. However, many of you likely focused on recording what was said, either in quotes or paraphrases, and gave little consideration to the reader's interest or the reason for documenting the story. But ask yourself, if you were going to retell the story to your parents versus another friend, would you retell it the same way? What if you were going to tell the story to a superior at work versus a significant other? Hopefully, you can see how authors, like speakers, need to self-regulate what information is communicated depending on their audience, purpose, and context for the situation. The problem for healthcare providers–authors involves the fact that the documents they create may be used by a breadth of readers—some peers, some superiors, and others including payers and lawyers—therefore, providers–authors need to understand as much as possible about the audience, purpose, and use for each patient record being created.

As we begin to discuss how to write patient records, it is important to recognize that the primary reason to write any type of document is to communicate information to a reader. Based on that understanding, healthcare providers–authors should recognize the importance of creating patient records that convey what the author intends to communicate and what the reader needs to properly use the document. Therefore, to write effective patient records, authors will benefit from an understanding of the basic principles of the writing process. In Chapter 1, we briefly discussed the various audiences, purposes, and uses for today's patient records. Understanding these components is critical to several stages of the writing process. This process is designed to help all types of authors identify, assess, and meet or surpass their readers' needs and expectations.

You may recall learning the writing process in your college composition courses. In order to review how critical the process is to authoring patient records, we need to examine some preliminary analyses that need to be undertaken prior to creating any patient record. Gurak and Lannon (2004), Heifferon (2005), Johnson-Eilola and Selber (2004), Pagano and Jacocks (1992), and Pagano and Ragan (1992) all discuss how these analyses need to include an understanding of the document's audience, purpose, and use.

Can you list potential readers of a patient record beyond those discussed in Chapter 1?

_____

_____

_____

Audience

Let us begin our discussion of the audience for patient records by exploring the potential members of that audience. Today, patient records are frequently used by every type of health care provider: MDs, DOs, RNs, PAs, APRNs, pharmacists, physical therapists, radiology technicians, social workers, and others. In addition, many patient records are also utilized by healthcare administrators, quality control regulators, insurance case managers, and attorneys. Therefore, before a provider authors a patient record, he or she needs to understand what these potential multiple readers' expectations are for the records they are reading.

Why do authors of scientific journal articles carefully document their research methods and their results?

_____

_____

_____

In all areas of scientific communication, we expect replication for validation (Keyton, 2006; Lyken, 1968). Consequently, readers of research want to know exactly how the research was conducted and what the specific findings were. Health care is no different. While it may not be the case that each reader of a patient record will be trying to physically replicate what the record's author heard, saw, and deduced, it is nonetheless a reality that almost all readers need sufficient information to virtually and intellectually replicate the author's discussion, examination, and decision making. So, the more you as an author of patient records can apply the concept of replication for validation to your communication, the more effective you will be. Armed with this understanding of what readers need to replicate your interaction with, and treatment of, a patient, let us discuss some specifics related to your audience, the purpose of the document you are creating, and how it is intended to be used.

In Chapter 1, you wrote a synopsis of an interaction with a friend. This is an example of many communication settings that occur in health care. In this culture, Americans like to use narratives to tell stories about their experiences. It is how they make sense of our world. Therefore, it is only natural that when Americans are ill or injured, they like to use a narrative to describe their situation, events, symptoms, and responses to prior treatment (du Pré, 2005; Geist-Martin, Ray & Sharf, 2003; Sharf & Vanderford, 2008). Similarly, providers need information from patients to assess the problem, treatment plan, and recent events; and readers of patient records generally need the same background information (past and present medical history, social and family history, etc.) as the author. Therefore, the patient's narrative is critically important to the provider's assessment of the problem and, by definition, will also be important to a reader's assessment of the patient's complaint, response to treatment, and so forth, as well as the reader's evaluation of the provider's decision making, course of action, and the like.

Take-Away Message

Whatever information you need as the provider to assess a patient's history, complaints, responses to treatment or decisions, you can expect your audience to need as well.

To discuss audience analysis for patient records, let us list some of the potential readers for patient records, depending on your profession, the purpose and use for the patient record, and the context:

- Physicians
- Physician assistants
- Advanced practice registered nurses
- Registered nurses
- Licensed practical nurses

- Certified nurse assistants
- Physical therapists
- Pharmacists
- Other healthcare professionals
- Administrators
- The Joint Commission
- Professional licensing boards
- Malpractice attorneys
- The patient and/or his or her family

While this list is not necessarily all-encompassing, you should be able to see the vast differences in roles, titles, status, and healthcare education between the diverse members. Unfortunately, providers–authors frequently fail to take into account the breadth of potential readers, and minimize or ignore the communication of the patient's narrative or other specific interaction-related information. Perhaps, decades ago, when authors primarily used the patient record as a memory device, this was an acceptable approach to documentation. However, with today's multi-audience needs and expectations for patient records, a provider–author should consider how important it is to document in considerable detail what she or he was told by the patient and/or family member for readers' analyses of the patient's situation. Let us look at an example of a patient record and evaluate the provider–author's analysis of the audience and their needs and expectations.

History and Physical (H&P) #1

Chief Complaint: Broken ankle.

Present Illness: This is a 22-year-old white male from California who is up here to climb rocks. He was climbing by himself tonight and fell about 20 feet, breaking his right ankle. He then climbed a total of 1/2 mile out of the area to receive help. He was brought to this hospital by his landlord for further evaluation. He is an epileptic and takes 400 mg of Dilantin daily. His last dose was today, and he needs 200 mg this evening. His health is otherwise fine.

Physical Examination: Shows a 22-year-old white male appearing his stated age in obvious distress from his ankle fracture.

HEENT: Normal.

Chest: Clear.

Heart: In regular rhythm, no murmurs.

Abdominal Exam: Unremarkable.

Extremities: Examination shows a distorted right ankle. X-ray reveals a fracture–dislocation of the talus.

Assessment: Fracture–dislocation, right talus. Epilepsy.

Plan: Operative reduction and internal fixation via Dr. _____. Maintain Dilantin level.

QUESTIONS

1. For a reader who will be providing care for this patient, what would be your assessment of the communication effectiveness of this H&P? Be as specific and detailed as you can be.

_____

_____

_____

_____

_____

_____

2. Based on the documentation of the patient's narrative, what information do you think is missing that a reader expects or needs to know to assess the patient's condition? Be as specific and detailed as possible.

_____

_____

_____

_____

_____

3. Since the patient fell 20 feet while climbing rocks, what are the top three questions you, as a reader, would want answers to?

_____

_____

_____

_____

_____

4. The H&P documents an x-ray report. What other tests, based on this patient's mechanism of injury—falling 20 feet while climbing rocks—would you want to know to determine if surgery is the appropriate next step? Why? Be as specific as possible.

_____

_____

_____

_____

_____

_____

5. Now that you have assessed an example of one provider's authoring of a patient record, what have you discovered about the role audience analysis plays in creating or reviewing healthcare documentation (in terms of the author's credibility, competence, diagnostic skills, malpractice risks, and so forth)?

_____

_____

_____

_____

_____

_____

_____

While it is true that this is only one example, it is, nonetheless, an actual patient record and not unique or atypical from a great deal of patient documentation. The problem for providers–authors is not recognizing the vital role that patient records play in health communication, reimbursement, and malpractice litigation. Healthcare providers are educated very thoroughly about the information, exams, diagnostic tests, and treatments needed to care for patients. However, what is frequently missing is an attention to the documentation of each of those aspects of patient care. And documenting conversations, exams, and tests does not mean supplying only the information that the provider feels is needed. Instead, documentation needs to include the information that a reader needs to arrive at the same assessment as the provider. As mentioned earlier, researchers are expected to provide the information needed to replicate studies. This same approach is a good way for providers–authors to think about their audience and how the patient record will be read and assessed. Providers–authors should ask themselves, what does the reader need to know in order to assess and concur with the authors' decision making? The more detailed and objective the data presented in the records, the easier it is for a reader to assess and evaluate the patient's complaints, condition, or treatment. Conversely, the more subjective (from the author's perspective) the information presented, the more difficult it is for a reader to assess and agree. Therefore, quotes from a patient, results of diagnostic tests, and a discussion of the critical thinking underlying an author's decision making are all very persuasive to readers. But providers–authors need to do more than just analyze their audience.

Purpose

While it is very important for providers–authors to assess the potential audience for their records, it is equally necessary for them to understand the purpose for creating each specific patient document. And even though the primary reason to author a patient record might seem obvious, there are a number of other factors that impact the purpose for creating a specific document.

> **When you think about patient records, what do you think are the major reasons for authoring them?**
>
> _____
>
> _____
>
> _____

There are numerous purposes for creating a patient record. Among the most critical are communicating the following:

- Patient's complaints, condition, or problems
- Provider's examination or intervention
- Diagnostic tests
- Provider's assessment of collected data
- Treatment plan decision-making process
- Responses to treatment

However, there are other purposes for authoring a patient document that include the following:

- Enhancing the provider–author's credibility with the reader
- Meeting organization and licensure requirements
- Communicating information needed for reimbursement
- Minimizing malpractice risk

These multiple purposes make authoring patient records much more difficult than many other forms of written communication. Therefore, let us examine how these diverse purposes impact the way you read a patient record. Please review an example of a discharge summary for the patient in H&P #1.

What do you think is important to include in a discharge summary in order to achieve the provider–author's purpose in creating the document?

_____

_____

_____

Discharge Summary #1

Admitted: 9/8/04

Discharged: 9/12/04

Admitting Diagnosis: Fracture–dislocation of the talus of the right foot.

Discharge Diagnosis: Same.

Brief History: 27-year-old male who was climbing rocks, fell about 15 feet, suffered a fracture–dislocation of his talus of this right foot. Physical examination was normal except for the ankle. X-rays revealed a fracture–dislocation of the talus.

Hospital Course: The patient was taken to the operating room and had an operative reduction, internal fixation of the talus. Postoperatively he had no problems. He will be discharged to continue on Tylenol #3 for pain and to see Dr. _____ in follow-up in 2 to 3 days.

QUESTIONS

1. Look at your answer to the last Q&A. Does this document meet your expectations for the provider–author's purpose(s)? If so, how? If not, why not? Be as specific and detailed as you can.

_____

_____

_____

_____

_____

2. If one of the author's purposes should be to illustrate his or her expertise and credibility, does this discharge summary positively or negatively impact those attributes? Compare to H&P #1 and be as specific and detailed as possible.

_____

_____

_____

_____

_____

_____

_____

3. For a healthcare reader, what information about the patient's hospitalization and discharge is missing that is needed to assess the patient's care and treatment?

_____

_____

_____

_____

_____

4. If this document is intended to be a summary of the patient's reason for hospitalization, treatment, response to treatment or outcome, and posthospitalization plan, does this patient record fulfill these goals? If yes, how? If no, why not? Be as specific as possible.

_____

_____

_____

_____

_____

_____

_____

5. If you were a malpractice attorney, either for the defense (author) or the plaintiff (patient), what would you find positive and negative in this document as it relates to the providers of this patient's care? Be as specific and detailed as possible.

_____

_____

_____

_____

_____

_____

_____

Do you think the author of H&P #1 and Discharge Summary #2 considered the multiple purposes for either of these documents prior to or after creating them? Why or why not?

_____

_____

_____

The purpose(s) for any patient record needs to be carefully considered _before_ the document is created. Then, the author should analyze the record after it has been completed to ensure that her or his intended goals and the readers' expectations and needs are both realized or surpassed. However, in addition to the audience and purpose analyses for any patient record, providers–authors need to consider how they intend the document to be used by the various readers.

Use

As important as it is to analyze an audience and the purpose for a patient record, it is equally critical to understand how you want a reader to use the document. For example, if you were creating a set of discharge instructions for a patient, you might want the patient to use the document to aid in compliance with agreed upon treatment plans. In addition, you might intend for those instructions to be used by members of the institution as fulfillment of the Joint Commission regulations (2009). Similarly, the author would likely want a colleague to find the instructions appropriate and similar to the standard of care for similar diseases or injuries. Healthcare professionals generally want their diverse audiences to use the patient records they create for the following:

- As the prime source for patient-related healthcare information
- To assess the provider–author's critical thinking
- To determine the credibility of the provider–author
- To evaluate the treatment decision making
- To determine the appropriateness of the care provided
- To minimize any malpractice risk
- To reimburse appropriately

Armed with these potential uses for any patient record, let us look at an example and analyze whether the document meets the potential uses a provider–author may have for such a record.

Chest X-Ray Report

Radiograph of the Chest: 02/02/06

Clinical Indication: Assess for pneumonia.

Technique: PA and lateral views of the chest with comparison to 1/19/06.

Findings: The cardiac silhouette and pulmonary vessels are within normal limits. There is no hilar or mediastinal adenopathy. Lungs are clear bilaterally. There is no effusion or pneumothorax. Visualized bones appear unremarkable.

Impression: No radiograph of the chest.

Reported and signed by: _____ , MD, 02/04/2006

QUESTIONS

1. How do you think the doctor–author of this chest x-ray report intended for it to be used by readers?

   _____

   _____

   _____

   _____

   _____

2. How does the author's communication of the findings and his or her impression change your evaluation of the author's ability and credibility? Be specific in detailing why you feel the way you do.

   _____

   _____

   _____

   _____

   _____

   _____

   _____

   _____

3. If you received this report, how would you use it to determine your patient's condition?

   _____

   _____

   _____

   _____

4. If the author of this document was involved in a malpractice case, how might this report be used against him or her?

   _____

   _____

   _____

   _____

_____

_____

_____

_____

5. What role does credibility play in your analysis of your written documents and the communication of your message?

   _____

   _____

   _____

   _____

   _____

   _____

   _____

The point is that the use for each and every patient record, regardless of whether it is authored in a hospital, outpatient, long-term care, rehabilitation, or private practice setting, needs to be clearly defined and understood by the provider–author. As we have just seen with the chest x-ray report, a document can include a wealth of information, but a miscommunication can confound and confuse a reader so much that she or he does not know what to believe in the report. If you got this report for a patient you were evaluating, would you not have to call the radiologist for a clarification? So, the audience, purpose, and use this document should have been created to address were all negatively impacted by the author's misstatement and absence, or poor quality, of proof-reading prior to signing and disseminating the patient record. The importance of analyzing your audience, purpose, and use for every document cannot be understated, but it will only be helpful if you revise and proofread your writing based on the decision making from your audience, purpose, and use analysis.

How might the audience, purposes, and uses be different for a Nurse's Note from a cardiac arrest in the emergency department (ED) versus routine care for a postpartum patient?

_____

_____

_____

This chapter has explored the importance of the provider–authors' understanding and analyzing of the audience, purpose, and use for every patient record. However, the context or setting, for any event has a major impact on your potential audience, purpose, and use for any document. For example, if you are involved in the resuscitation of a patient in the ED following a cardiac arrest, your audience will expect your documentation to be much more detailed and specific than if you were authoring a Nurse's Note for a patient who had a routine vaginal delivery of a healthy full-term infant. And while that may seem commonsensical, the reality of life in contemporary American healthcare organizations is that many authors, like those in the three examples in this chapter, do not communicate effectively in their patient records and consequently cause problems for their readers, as well as credibility and potential malpractice issues for themselves.

Skills Application

You are working in a hospital and need to write a patient record (appropriate for your profession) for a patient who had some type of intervention, treatment, or therapy that was not successful or effective. The patient had a poor outcome.

1. Analyze who your audience would be for this record. Be as specific as possible.

   _____

   _____

   _____

   _____

   _____

2. Analyze the purpose(s) for which you are authoring this record. Be as detailed as possible.

   _____

   _____

   _____

   _____

   _____

3. Assess how you want this document to be used by your audience.

In Chapter 3, we will explore the writing process you may want to adapt so you can quickly and efficiently analyze your audience, purpose, and use for any patient record you author. This authoring process will provide you with a method that addresses the results of your analysis and affords you an opportunity to assess and revise your document to make it more effective and useful for readers.

REFERENCES

du Pré, A. (2005). *Communicating about health: Current issues and perspectives* (2nd ed.). Boston, MA: McGraw-Hill.

Geist-Martin, P., Ray, E., & Sharf, B. (2003). *Communicating health: Personal, cultural, and political complexities*. Belmont, CA: Thomson/Wadsworth.

Gurak, L., & Lannon, J. (2004). *A concise guide to technical communication* (2nd ed.). New York, NY: Pearson-Longman.

Heifferon, B. (2005). *Writing in the health professions*. New York, NY: Pearson-Longman.

Johnson-Eilola, J., & Selber, S. (2004). *Central works in technical communication*. New York, NY: Oxford University Press.

Joint Commission on Accreditation of Healthcare Organizations (2009). Retrieved on January 20, 2009, from http://www.jointcommission.org/.

Keyton, J. (2006). *Communication research: Asking questions, finding answers*. Boston: McGraw-Hill.

Lyken, D. (1968). Statistical significance in psychological research. *Psychological Bulletin, 70,* 151–159.

Pagano, M., & Jacocks, M. (1992). *Communicating effectively in medical records: A guide for physicians*. Newbury Park, CA: Sage.

Pagano, M., & Ragan, S. (1992). *Communication skills for professional nurses*. Newbury Park, CA: Sage.

Sharf, B., & Vanderford, M. (2008). Illness narratives and social construction of health. In L. C. Lederman (Ed.), *Beyond these walls: Readings in health communication* (pp. 24–46). New York, NY: Oxford University Press.

Chapter 3

Developing an Authoring Process

Overview

The purpose of this chapter is to help you develop a process for authoring patient records. This book uses the term *authoring* as opposed to writing because not all patient records are written in the traditional sense of that word. Today, health-care providers write some documents, but they also create electronic documents, complete templates and/or checklists, and dictate some patient records (Häyrinen, Saranto, & Nykänen, 2008; Heifferon, 2005; Pagano, 2009). Compared to 50 years ago, when the majority of all patient records were actually written in ink, today, there are numerous formats (written, dictated, checklists, electronic, and so forth) for conveying patient-related health communication. Therefore, a provider–author needs to have a process that will assist her or him with developing and documenting the necessary information to communicate with an audience, regardless of the format used to create the record.

Traditionally, in academic, scientific, and professional writing courses, the process has been divided into four diverse but interrelated and interdependent steps: pre-authoring, authoring, revising–reviewing, and proofreading (Gurak & Lannon, 2004; Pagano & Jacocks, 1992; Pagano & Ragan, 1992). This chapter will discuss each of these steps and how they can assist you in creating more effective patient records. However, learning a process for authoring patient records will only be beneficial if it can accomplish a provider–author's multiple goals. Therefore, to be successful, this authoring process must be effective for the following:

- Any type of patient record
- All healthcare professionals' needs
- Every format for creating a patient care document
- Diverse provider–authors' goals
- A breadth of audiences, purposes, and uses

Authoring patient records is a legally required, time-consuming, communication skill that all healthcare providers must master as part of their clinical training. However, for too many providers, this skill has not been taught using a process model, is minimally practiced, and has not been assessed to the same extent as other clinical skills. Instead, authoring patient documents is frequently relegated to self-learning, or apprentice work, through trial and error based on mimicking examples of other providers' records. As we know from other professions, there are enormous risks associated with this type of pedagogy.

As you no doubt have surmised, learning any skill by copying someone else's example is fraught with risk. Primarily, the student's ability to learn a skill in this manner is totally dependent upon the effectiveness of the example being imitated and the communication assessment capability of the mentor–instructor who chose the example and evaluates the students' work. Consequently, healthcare providers–authors would be much better served if they could learn a self-directed process for authoring patient records that educated them about the audience's needs and expectations, as well as the multiple purposes and uses for the various documents. And, even more valuable would be a process that helps providers–authors use critical thinking to analyze the current setting and situation and to create the most effective communication to meet or exceed the audience's requirements or expectations for such a document. This chapter will help you learn such a process, and while it may require some extra time at the outset to learn and practice the skill, like all skills, with increased practice and use you will become faster and more effective as you progress and master it.

> If you have to write a paper in a course, how do you start the process (what are steps one, two, and three, and why)?
> _____
> _____
> _____

The Blank Page

One of the most terrifying things for any author of an assignment is the sight of a blank page (paper or computer screen). Authoring, no matter whether you are a novelist, academic, scientist, copy writer, or healthcare professional, is an onerous task. Authors need to gather and assimilate information and then analyze what messages are necessary to communicate that information to an audience. In addition, authors must find an appropriate format and symbols (words and/or numbers) to communicate that information to an audience who likely may have different education levels, expectations, and needs than the author. For health-care providers, as compared to other types of authors, the information to be communicated in patient records is always patient-related, and the format for those documents is generally predetermined by the provider's profession and the purpose and/or use for the record being created.

Therefore, it might appear on first consideration to be much easier to author a patient document than other types of written communication, but the diverse audiences, purposes, and uses for patient records create a number of unique and potentially risky challenges. A physical therapist, for example, knows that her or his record of a patient's treatment will need to follow a set format and style; however, the information that needs to be included in such a record, both in quantity and specificity, is not necessarily predetermined. Instead, the expected information is based on a wide range of factors that must be assessed and critically analyzed by the physical therapist–author for each document in order to effectively meet both the author and the readers' needs and expectations for that particular patient record. For example, a patient who is improving with treatment will likely require a different set of communication symbols and discussion than one who is not improving, versus one who is getting worse or missing appointments. The point is that you as a provider–author do not want to start to create a patient record with a blank page; you want to have analyzed what is needed, based on the document, the patient, his or her situation, and the audience, purpose, and use for the record. By having pre-analyzed what needs to be communicated for each patient record that you author, you will save yourself time, more effectively communicate your information, and have a guide to use in assessing whether your document accomplishes the goals you intended.

Step One: Pre-Authoring

In order to avoid that dreaded blank page and to become faster at creating patient records, you need to start your communication process with *pre-authoring*. Pre-authoring, as the term implies, refers to the work you need to do prior to actually authoring any document. Pre-authoring can be done anywhere and does not necessarily require any actual writing or typing. Pre-authoring should include some very precise but not necessarily linear steps (many, if not all can be done concurrently):

1. Gather data (from a patient interaction, exam, or tests, etc.).
2. Use critical thinking to analyze which data are necessary for the particular patient's record based upon the following:
   - Expected audience
   - Anticipated purpose(s)
   - Intended uses
3. Determine the quantity and specificity of data needed to be communicated.

Pre-Authoring Audience Analysis

In Chapter 2 we discussed the importance of audience analysis. As you may recall, most patient records have both primary and secondary audiences. Primary audiences generally include other members of the healthcare team who need to know the patient-related information you have gathered. Some of the many possible primary audiences for a patient record include, but are not limited to, the following:

- Physicians
- Physician assistants
- Advanced practice registered nurses
- Registered nurses
- Licensed practical nurses
- Social workers
- Physical therapists
- Pharmacists
- Home health agencies
- Rehabilitation or long-term care facilities
- Healthcare insurers

As you can see, the majority of the primary audiences for most patient records are other healthcare providers; however, because reimbursement is critical to a patient's ability to seek medical care and to most providers' livelihoods, it can be argued that it is necessary to create patient records that meet the expectations and needs of healthcare insurers.

In analyzing the education and health literacy levels of the vast majority of primary audiences, medical terminology can be expected to be part of the author–audiences' shared symbols. In addition, the goals for most primary audiences and providers–authors should also be shared: improving or maintaining the patient's health and wellness. Therefore, providers–authors and primary audiences can be expected to share many of the same communication symbols, goals, and expectations. However, besides primary audiences, there are a number of secondary audiences who utilize patient records.

Secondary audiences have diverse purposes and uses for patient records. These secondary audiences may include the following:

- Hospital administrators
  - Quality care
  - Finance
  - Risk management
  - Infection control

- Government agencies
  - Centers for Disease Control and Prevention
  - State public health office
- Employers for workers' compensation cases
- Patients and/or family members
- Malpractice attorneys

Compared to the primary audiences, secondary audiences are much more diverse in their education levels, shared symbols, and goals. Clearly, a number of these possible readers–users of patient records may not understand medical terminology or share the same goals as the author. For example, most employers could be expected to want their employees back to work as soon as possible, while healthcare providers may be focusing on making sure an injury is completely healed first. The problem for authors of patient records is the ever-expanding secondary audience for patient records and the decreasing time available to create and review the documents.

Skills Application

1. Write a paragraph for college students that describes your healthcare profession.

_____

_____

_____

_____

_____

_____

QUESTIONS

1. How did you decide what information your college reader would want, expect, or need?

_____

_____

_____

_____

2. Did you spend any time determining if you needed to use different words
    to ensure your college reader's understanding? If yes, why? If no, why not?

    _____

    _____

Skills Application

1. Now write a paragraph about your profession, but this time author it to
    be read by a class of fourth graders.

    _____

    _____

    _____

    _____

    _____

    _____

QUESTIONS

1. How was authoring this paragraph for fourth graders different from the
    previous one for college students? Be very specific and detailed.

    _____

    _____

    _____

    _____

2. Did you spend any time determining if you needed to use different words
    to ensure your fourth-grade reader's understanding? If yes, why? If no,
    why not?

    _____

    _____

    _____

    _____

    _____

This exercise is intended to illustrate the difficulties for an author based on a single change—the education level of the audience. Please note how much more difficult this could have been if the document for fourth graders had to be two pages instead of one paragraph. Or, what if you had an additional purpose for authoring the fourth-graders' paragraph—to get the school to pay you for your work? This seemingly simple task of authoring a document about a topic that is very well known by you becomes so much more difficult based on the audience and their literacy levels. Hopefully, you can begin to see the problem for a provider–author based solely on the diverse audiences for patient records and their diverse education, health literacy, and healthcare backgrounds. However, in addition to the potential problems presented by audiences of patient records, the purpose(s) for each patient document created by a provider–author needs to be thoroughly analyzed and explored.

Pre-Authoring Purpose Analysis

Chapter 2 discussed the various purposes for patient records in some detail, but providers–authors need to spend a little time analyzing the potential purpose(s) for every patient document. In this chapter, we want to understand how those multipurposes impact your pre-authoring analyses and decision making. Let us look at an example to see how numerous issues can alter the purposes of a document. You have a patient who is otherwise healthy but hit his head and feels dizzy, but did not lose consciousness. You have another patient who is healthy and needs an annual exam. Your third patient hit her hand, you read her hand x-ray as negative, and she has no other complaints or problems.

Skills Application

1. For the patient who hit his head and feels dizzy, but did not lose consciousness, what are your top three purposes for authoring a patient record and why?

   _____

   _____

   _____

   _____

   _____

   _____

2. For the healthy patient who needs an annual exam, what are your top three purposes for authoring a patient record and why?

   _____

   _____

   _____

   _____

3. For the patient who hit her hand, and you read her x-ray as negative, what are your top three purposes for authoring a patient record and why?

   _____

   _____

   _____

   _____

   _____

4. In your analyses of these three different patients and their patient records, what did you find similar, different, and thought provoking? Try to be as reflective and detailed as possible.

   _____

   _____

   _____

   _____

   _____

   _____

As you no doubt surmised, there are some obvious similarities in terms of the purpose for patient records regardless of the patient, his or her problem or reason for the visit, or the type of document; however, there are some very important differences as well. For example, one of the major purposes for authoring a patient record for each of these three patients is to communicate information about them and their visit or problem; however, that purpose will dictate in some ways the quantity of information needed for each. The head trauma patient will need very specific and detailed information related to his injury, his postinjury mental status, and your physical exam findings, test results, and so forth. The record of the annual physical exam will require more diverse information about the patient's past, present, family, and social histories, as well as a discussion of a complete physical exam and all laboratory, electrocardiogram, x-ray, or other tests.

The final patient will likely have the most focused and limited discussion of information related to her injury, the exam of her hand, her x-ray, and treatment plan. Therefore, even though a major purpose—communicating information—is the same for each of these patient records for the three patients, the content to fulfill all the purposes for authoring them will be vastly different.

A second major purpose for these three patient records is to demonstrate to readers that the provider–author did an appropriate patient interview and exam. By communicating this information in the document, the author is expecting that his or her ability to assess and treat the patient will not be called into question by the primary or secondary audiences. Therefore, it will be very important for the provider–author of the patient record for the head trauma patient to document the patient's mechanism of injury; mental status; head, eyes, ears, nose, mouth, and neck exam; as well as communicating in the patent record a detailed neurologic and musculoskeletal evaluation, plus any tests and the course of treatment. The provider–author wants to anticipate her or his audience's questions and answer them in the document as if readers were interviewing and examining the head injury patient themselves.

Similarly, a third major purpose for authoring these three patient records might be to enhance the provider–author's credibility with primary and secondary readers, thus reinforcing the reader's acceptance of, or concurrence with, the provider–author's information, decision making, and treatment plans or actions. This purpose is important for the provider–author from a standard of care, economic reimbursement, and medical and legal perspectives.

Providers–authors need to recognize that patient records may have different purposes, based on a number of factors such as the reason for the provider–patient interaction, the patient's problem or condition, the provider's analysis of the situation, decision making, and/or treatments (next steps). While it is true that all patient records share one major purpose—to communicate information about a particular patient—it is also true that most patient records have diverse other purposes, and these need to be assessed and addressed by the provider–author in his or her documentation to ensure that all of the patient record's purposes are fulfilled and effectively communicated to the primary and secondary audiences.

To better understand how the audience and purpose for patient records impact readers' evaluations, let us revisit H&P #1. Try and assess whether or not you think the provider–author of this document did any pre-authoring related to the audiences and purposes for this particular patient's record.

History and Physical (H&P) #1

Chief Complaint: Broken ankle.

Present Illness: This is a 22-year-old white male from California who is up here to climb rocks. He was climbing by himself tonight and fell about 20 feet, breaking his right ankle. He then climbed a total of 1/2 mile out of the area to receive help. He was brought to this hospital by his landlord for further evaluation. He is an epileptic and takes 400 mg of Dilantin daily. His last dose was today, and he needs 200 mg this evening. His health is otherwise fine.

Physical Examination: Shows a 22-year-old white male appearing his stated age in obvious distress from his ankle fracture.

HEENT: Normal.

Chest: Clear.

Heart: In regular rhythm, no murmurs.

Abdominal Exam: Unremarkable.

Extremities: Examination shows a distorted right ankle. X-ray reveals a fracture–dislocation of the talus.

Assessment: Fracture–dislocation, right talus. Epilepsy.

Plan: Operative reduction and internal fixation via Dr. _____. Maintain Dilantin level.

QUESTIONS

1. What do you think are the purposes for authoring this patient record?

   _____

   _____

   _____

   _____

2. Does the record address the purposes you identified? If yes, how? If no, why not?

   _____

   _____

   _____

   _____

3. If you were the author of this patient record, is there any additional information you think the primary and/or secondary readers might need–expect? Why, or why not?

_____

_____

_____

_____

As secondary readers for H&P #1 and healthcare professionals, we likely can see some possible issues with the way this document communicates information (one of its primary purposes). For example, how does the document communicate the provider–patient interaction and examination? As documented in the record, how do you assess the provider–author's professional ability and credibility? Let us look at what the author chooses to communicate about the patient who fell 20 feet while climbing rocks. As a healthcare reader, one of the first questions you might want answered by the provider–author for this patient is, did the patient hit his head or lose consciousness in a 20-foot fall on rocky terrain? Your expectation would likely be that there is a very high probability that a fall from that height in rocks would entail some head trauma accompanying an ankle fracture. In addition, if there is a risk of head injury, then there is an equally strong possibility of cervical trauma, and yet, there is no record of a discussion with the patient about head or neck trauma, or even loss of consciousness.

In addition, a fall from such a height carries a high risk of thoracic and abdominal injuries, either of which could cause major problems intraoperatively, and yet, there is no mention of any abrasions, lacerations, or hematomas anywhere on the body from a 20-foot fall in the rocks. By not mentioning the presence or absence of any skin wounds, the provider–author raises more questions for readers about the patient's exam and the author's expertise and abilities. Furthermore, there is no discussion of a computerized axial tomography (CAT) scan of the abdomen, or even a chest x-ray to rule out a pneumothorax. In fact, the entire provider–author's objective findings on the physical examination are 22 words in total. A patient falls 20 feet, fractures his ankle, crawls a half mile in rocky terrain, and is going to surgery, and the entire provider–author assessment of the physical examination findings is 22 words long. If this patient goes into shock or has a pneumothorax, an intracranial hemorrhage, or a neck injury intra- or postoperatively, how would the provider–author of H&P #1 ever be able to expect readers to find his interview, exam, analysis, decision making, and treatment plan appropriate to meet the standard of care for such a situation or patient?

As you may have determined, a provider–author who fails to meet the reader's needs and the purposes for which the patient record is intended does not communicate effectively and calls into question his or her assessment, diagnostic skills, and treatment decision making. The importance of pre-authoring is that providers can analyze, based on the patient and his or her situation, what information is critical and in what detail to meet the audience's needs and to fulfill the purposes for authoring the document. However, providers–authors also need to recognize the importance of how the document will be used in their pre-authoring analysis.

Pre-Authoring Use Analysis

As compared to audience and purpose analyses for your patient record, the evaluation of how a provider–author wants her or his record to be used is more predictable, but equally important to consider. For many situations, the provider–author will want the patient record to be used as fulfillment of a requirement or legal obligation to communicate information about a patient's examination and treatment. In addition, providers–authors want their records to be used as sources of information necessary to obtain reimbursement from health insurance companies. And, most records need to be used to illustrate and demonstrate the provider–author's professional ability, expertise, and credibility to minimize the risk of malpractice litigation.

As you read the following Nurse's Note for an obstetrical patient, consider how you would use this record if you were the provider–author's supervisor, a Joint Commission reviewer, or a malpractice attorney.

Nurse's Note

2200–   Patient had a contriction and rolled around on the bed until she fell to the floor. She didn't lose consciousness and she didn't complain of any pain, except in her gluteal area.

2230–   Dr. _____ and Dr. _____ in to see patient. Epidural anesthetic given. Patient's vital signs and fetal heart tone are ok.

2255–   Fully dilated; moved to Delivery.

2311–   Vaginal delivery of 9.2 pound boy with APGER of 9.

2335–   Mother and baby returned to Room 512. (Pagano & Ragan, 1992, p. 107)

This is an example of a signed patient record.

QUESTIONS

1. As you read this document, how did you assess the provider–author's understanding of how this record would be used by her or his supervisor, other providers, or a Joint Commission reviewer?

_____

_____

_____

_____

2. Do you think this document could be used to meet either the primary or secondary audiences' expectations or needs? If so, why? If not, why not?

_____

_____

_____

_____

3. What did you find troubling from a professional credibility and expertise perspective in the documentation of this patient's condition and situation? Why?

_____

_____

_____

_____

As you may have noticed, this Nurse's Note has a number of problems from a reader's perspective, as well as from the provider–author's viewpoint. The glaring issues related to the misspelled words ("contriction" instead of "contraction" and "APGER" instead of "APGAR") immediately call into question the provider–author's knowledge and thoroughness. That reality, coupled with the fact that the patient fell out of bed, with no discussion of the status of her bedrails, hematomas, abrasions, or specific vital signs and fetal heart tones prods a reader to question if the spelling errors are a hurried authoring miscue or an indication of this provider–author's lack of attention to detail or ineptitude. You can feel pretty certain that the provider–author of this simple document did not intend for it to be used to question his or her ability as a healthcare professional. Similarly, you would expect that the provider–author did not want her or his supervisor, peers, or the Joint Commission reviewers to use this record as an example of substandard documentation or even worse, substandard care. By not describing in far greater detail the patient's incident and the provider–author's response, assessment, and actions, readers are left to wonder about the nurse's expertise and the hospital's training and safety.

The apparent lack of pre-authoring analysis of the audience, purpose, and use for this record, coupled with the provider–author's paucity of revising and/or proofreading, highlights the onerous nature of authoring patient records. The value of pre-authoring the effective communication of information by healthcare providers cannot be minimized. However, far too few healthcare providers are ever taught an authoring process or the importance of pre-authoring, and consequently, their efforts to document appropriately and effectively are all too frequently similar to H&P #1 and the Nurse's Note above.

Step Two: Authoring

The authoring process as we have discussed has four distinct phases that are interrelated and interdependent. As we have just explored, pre-authoring is very important for a provider–author's understanding of the audience's needs, purposes, and uses for every patient record. Pre-authoring, however, often requires no actual writing or typing. A provider–author, over time and with practice, may become adept at quickly assessing his or her audience, purposes, and uses for the particular patient document being created. However, with more complicated contexts and unexpected outcomes, providers–authors might want to quickly jot down the key points that need to be addressed, areas to be supported, direct quotes, objective findings, and so forth, to ensure that they are communicated in the finished patient record.

Conversely, the authoring phase of the process is defined by the need to actually put words into a document related to the topic being communicated. In other types of writing—scholarly, academic, scientific, business—this phase of the process is generally considered to be less structured and more creative in the sense that the writer is trying to get her or his ideas on paper without worrying about the rules for authoring, grammar, and style. However, in creating patient records, providers generally focus the overwhelming majority of their efforts on this *authoring* phase of the process.

Whereas authors in other fields may spend more time on pre-authoring and re-authoring than on the actual authoring phase of the process, for healthcare providers the authoring phase tends to dominate the process. This reality is critical to improving your patient records. Providers–authors frequently point to time constraints, the repetitive nature of medical documents, provider–patient interaction, and other administrative duties as reasons for not spending more time on pre-authoring, re-authoring, and/or proofreading. Therefore, it is not uncommon for a student–provider to be taught to author patient records using an apprentice model in which the student is given a document and told to follow it as a template for the record she or he is creating. In this model, the emphasis is immediately placed on the authoring that is included, or missing, from the template document. There is no understanding or analysis of the template or the author's pre-authoring or re-authoring decision making. The template becomes the model for the student–author's documentation and eliminates any sense of an interrelated and interdependent, iterative process.

Effective written communication generally results from the interplay between what an author wants to convey to readers, what a document actually communicates, and how the document can be revised to better meet the author's pre-authoring goals and objectives and the readers' needs and expectations. This nonlinear, iterative process examines the author's intended message for a specific audience, purpose, and use, with the message being communicated by the created document, and uses critical analysis to constantly reassess the original goals and ideas with the latest stage–draft of the authored record.

Consequently, had the provider–author of H&P #1 used the authoring process in the traditional way it is taught and practiced, he or she would have written a draft and read the H&P and compared it to his or her pre-authoring analysis. Such an evaluation would have likely resulted in the provider–author's recognition that the document needed re-authoring to accomplish the provider–author's intended purposes and uses for the patient record. This is the traditional method many authors use to organize their message, communicate it, analyze it, reshape it, reanalyze it, and so on. However, as mentioned above, this is not typical of most provider–authors' documentation processes. The goal of this book is to help you see the value of the authoring process and to encourage you to learn these skills. The more you practice them, the faster you will get at using them, and the more effective your patient record communication will become.

> Can you recall a time when you had a professor, parent, or friend read something you had written and provided you with feedback? If so, what did you do with that person's suggestions and recommendations?
>
> _____
>
> _____
>
> _____

Step Three: Re-Authoring

If you are like most current or former college students, you have authored a paper that had to be submitted to a professor who read it, provided feedback, and asked you to rewrite it. If so, then you have practiced the skill of re-authoring. However, for most postgraduate authors, this process is not related to a third-person respondent, but instead to the author's own analysis of the document, created and a comparison to some virtual or written audience analyses, goals, messages, purposes, and uses. The value of comparing what a document communicates to what the author intended it to convey is critical to effectively sharing information, minimizing confusion, and eliminating miscommunication. As you know, one of the major differences between written (hand or electronic) communication and face-to-face interaction is the absence of feedback from the audience.

> List some examples of verbal and nonverbal feedback you use to determine if your face-to-face message has been effectively communicated or has confused an individual or audience.
>
> _____
>
> _____
>
> _____

In lieu of verbal or nonverbal feedback for their written communication, authors must rely on their own postauthoring analysis of the effectiveness, information sharing, and clarity of their documents; however, this process depends on a provider–author reviewing her or his record and revising it. Unfortunately, far too many provider–authors do not understand the importance of this step in the authoring process or do not take the time to review the document prior to signing it.

Let us revisit the Nurse's Note discussed earlier in this chapter.

Nurse's Note

2200– Patient had a contriction and rolled around on the bed until she fell to the floor. She didn't lose consciousness and she didn't complain of any pain, except in her gluteal area.

2230– Dr. _____ and Dr. _____ in to see patient. Epidural anesthetic given. Patient's vital signs and fetal heart tone are ok.

2255– Fully dilated; moved to Delivery.

2311– Vaginal delivery of 9.2 pound both with APGER of 9.

2335– Mother and baby returned to Room 512. (Pagano & Ragan, 1992, p. 107)

If you were the provider–author of this document and, prior to signing it, you read over it and considered your pre-authoring assessment of the audience, purposes, and uses for this document, you could have rewritten it to better meet those pre-authoring goals and objectives. For example, the provider–author might have rewritten the first portion of the document for this patient.

Nurse's Notes (Revised)

2200– Ms. _____ was having contractions about 2 minutes apart. The fetal heart rate was 148. The patient had an apparent contraction, and, while screaming in pain, she rolled abruptly onto her left side and struck the raised side rail. However, the side rail broke, and the patient rolled about 2 feet from the bed to the floor. She landed on her gluteus and did not strike her head, neck, or abdomen. I was standing a few feet from her. She had no loss of consciousness. I asked her if she had any pain and she replied, "No, just my butt hurts."

I pressed the emergency buzzer, asked the patient to stay on the floor until two other nurses _____ and _____ arrived to help me get the patient back into bed. Ms. _____'s vital signs after the fall were: pulse 98, respiration 14, and blood pressure 132/88. These results compared with P. 88, R. 14, and BP. 118/72 taken 10 minutes before the fall. The fetal heart tone was 148 after the fall and unchanged compared to before. Her lung sounds were clear after the fall. Her right gluteus was red, but there was no hematoma, laceration, or abrasion. An ice bag was applied to the area. I notified Dr. _____ of the incident and the patient's condition. Dr. _____ had no new orders. I notified _____, the Labor and Delivery Supervisor on duty and completed an incident report.

QUESTIONS

1. How would you compare this entry for 2200 hours to the previous one in terms of the audience, purpose, and use analysis for such a document? Please be detailed in your discussion of your response to the two records.

   _____

   _____

   _____

   _____

   _____

   _____

2. Why do you think this rewrite contains the specific names of the nurses who came to help after the fall?

_____

_____

_____

3. Do you think this level of detail would be necessary for this OB patient's notes if she had not fallen? Why do you feel that way?

_____

_____

_____

Would the revision example shown here have taken more time than the original Nurse's Note? Absolutely. It would have taken a couple of minutes longer, but look at the advantages and benefits for the provider–author from taking those extra few minutes.

- A reader knows exactly what happened.
- There is no question about the prefall status of the bed rails.
- The provider–author's status during the event is clearly documented.
- Objective data are supplied to help readers analyze the postfall situation and the patient's condition; the provider–author did not rely on subjective statements "she didn't complain of any pain."
- Readers' questions are answered by the revised documentation.
- The provider–author's skills, expertise, and credibility are enhanced.

As you can tell, both of these examples are selections from a patient's Nurse's Notes. But, the former raises more questions for both primary and secondary readers than it answers and, thus, fails to achieve even the most basic purpose for authoring it: sharing information. The point of this discussion is that providers–authors can spend a few minutes analyzing a record they created and revising it, or they can risk the problems that may come from ineffective communication or miscommunication in a patient document.

By using the authoring process, providers–authors can identify for themselves the information they need to communicate, how it should be presented, and in what detail and clarification. Then, they can analyze the documents they create using the material from their pre-authoring to determine where revisions need to be made to ensure that the patient record more effectively and clearly meets both the provider–author's and the reader's needs and expectations as well as the purpose(s) for authoring it.

Have you ever created a budget? If so, then you know that a budget is your plan for how much you want to spend on various items or categories. But, to make a budget truly effective and reflective of your spending versus your goals, what do you need to do on a regular basis?

_____

_____

_____

Thus far, we have examined an H&P, Discharge Summary, and Nurse's Notes and have seen how the providers–authors for these various documents either did not use pre-authoring and re-authoring or did not do it effectively. The result of those omissions or shortcomings are patient records that do not communicate as intended or call into question the provider–author's intelligence, experience, diagnostic and communication skills, and/or credibility. You as a provider–author can choose to utilize the authoring process to help you enhance your patient records and their communication effectiveness, or not. However, even if you choose to use the process and pre-author, author, and re-author, there is one step that remains to be completely effective.

Step Four: Proofreading

You have taken the time to analyze your audience, purposes, and uses for the document you are creating, and you have assessed the document to determine where it meets your pre-authoring goals and objectives and where it needs work, and you have made those changes. So, are you done? No, not quite. There is one more step before you sign the record and make it a legal document— you need to proofread it.

Re-authoring is the act of reviewing the content of a document to determine how it meets the provider's pre-authoring analysis of what is necessary to communicate to the audience. Proofreading, on the other hand, is carefully reading through the document to make sure there are no missing words, misspelled words, typos (for example "there" instead of "their"), or grammatical miscues. While you as a provider–author may think this is a silly step in the process, I would like to remind you of the chest x-ray report from Chapter 2 that was a signed, legal document.

Chest X-Ray Report

Radiograph of the Chest: 02/02/06

Clinical Indication: Assess for pneumonia.

Technique: PA and lateral views of the chest with comparison to 1/19/06.

Findings: The cardiac silhouette and pulmonary vessels are within normal limits. There is no hilar or mediastinal adenopathy. Lungs are clear bilaterally. There is no effusion or pneumothorax. Visualized bones appear unremarkable.

Impression: No radiograph of the chest.

Reported and signed by: _____, MD, 02/04/2006

Here, we have an example of a patient record that the provider–author, a radiologist, dictated and then signed. The provider–author is responsible for this document, so it does not matter who made the mistake (transcriptionist or provider) "No radiograph of the chest." It is the author who signed the record who is legally responsible for any mistakes. Had the radiologist taken the time to read over this record, prior to signing it, she or he hopefully would have found this mistake (perhaps a typo, perhaps a misstatement when dictating) and could have easily corrected it, prior to signing. However, because it was not corrected, both the primary and secondary audiences for this record may question the provider–author's skills, expertise, and especially his or her thoroughness.

As a radiologist, who is expected to critically and meticulously review radiographs and scans, do you think the provider–author wants to call into question his or her skill or thoroughness? It would seem very unlikely that a provider–author would desire such additional consternation. However, a signed, legal record that has such an obvious mistake in the specialist's interpretation of the test creates enormous potential problems for the provider–author.

Proofreading patient records—whether they are handwritten, transcribed, or electronically created—takes very little time, but offers enormous potential rewards. Providers–authors need to recognize the problems created by patient documents that do not illustrate the author's observation and analytical skills, as well as her or his attention to detail. By critically proofreading a patient record prior to signing it and ensuring there are no missing or misspelled words, typos, or grammatical errors, providers–authors can enhance their credibility with their audience and positively impact a document's purpose and use.

The four steps of the authoring process can, with practice and experience, be done in very little time. However, providers–authors need to recognize the important role that this process plays in patient documentation, provider credibility, and malpractice risk reduction. Learning, practicing, and adopting the authoring process to your authoring of patient records will reap you vast rewards and enhance both your professional stature and your patients' care.

REFERENCES

Gurak, L., & Lannon, J. (2004). *A concise guide to technical communication* (2nd ed.). New York, NY: Pearson-Longman.

Häyrinen, K., Saranto, K., & Nykänen, P. (2008). Definition, structure, content, use, and impacts of electronic health records: A review of the research literature. *International Journal of Medical Informatics.*

Heifferon, B. (2005). *Authoring in the health professions*. New York, NY: Pearson-Longman.

Pagano, M. (2009). *Converting to an electronic patient record: Dialectics of organizational change.* Manuscript submitted for publication.

Pagano, M., & Jacocks, M. (1992). *Communicating effectively in patient records: A guide for physicians.* Newbury Park, CA: Sage.

Pagano, M., & Ragan, S. (1992). *Communication skills for professional nurses.* Newbury Park, CA: Sage.

Chapter 4

Adapting the Reporter's Formula

Who's on First

Bud Abbott and Lou Costello had a comedy routine based around a baseball question–statement of "who's on first." They went back and forth about Who was on first and What being on second, and so on. The joke was that the players' names were Who and What, but Costello thought Abbott was asking him the names of the players. Part of the routine included the following exchange:

Costello: Well then who's on first?
Abbott: Yes.
Costello: I mean the fellow's name.
Abbott: Who.
Costello: The guy on first.
Abbott: Who.
Costello: The first baseman.
Abbott: Who.
Costello: The guy playing . . .
Abbott: Who is on first!
Costello: I'm asking you who's on first.
Abbott: That's the man's name.
Costello: That's who's name?
Abbott: Yes.
Costello: Well go ahead and tell me.
Abbott: That's it.
Costello: That's who?
Abbott: Yes. PAUSE
Costello: Look, you gotta first baseman?
Abbott: Certainly.

Costello: Who's playing first?

Abbott: That's right.

Costello: When you pay off the first baseman every month, who gets the money?

Abbott: Every dollar of it.

Costello: All I'm trying to find out is the fellow's name on first base.

Abbott: Who.

Costello: The guy that gets . . .

Abbott: That's it. (Abbott & Costello, 2000, para. 5)

Why is this so funny that it is part of the Baseball Hall of Fame? How does it illustrate the confusion caused by a lack of detail and content?

_____

_____

_____

_____

This dialogue, while intended to be funny, points out the importance of effective communication and how content shapes an audience's understanding or confusion related to a message.

In the previous chapters, we have discussed how important the authoring process is to your documentation in patient records. Now, we need to explore how you can enhance the content of your documents to better meet the readers' needs and expectations and minimize or eliminate any confusion or questions. Journalists use a model to help them obtain as much information about a topic or from an interviewee as possible and to assess their authoring to ensure it communicates sufficient detail. This model is called the *Reporter's Formula* and includes a series of questions that are used to focus the author's exploration of a topic and to ensure broad coverage and analysis. Specifically, the Reporter's Formula seeks answers to the following questions:

1. Who?
2. What?
3. Where?
4. When?
5. Why?
6. How?

These six simple questions can assist providers–authors with obtaining the information they need for almost any patient documentation. At the same time, the formula provides authors a tool to aid in assessing the record created to ensure it communicates effectively the content an audience expects and needs. There is no order to how the questions should be asked, or even the context surrounding their use; that is generally determined by the project. However, the more you use the Reporter's Formula to focus and organize your information gathering and documentation, the better it will be for you as a healthcare provider, for your readers, and ultimately, for your patient's care.

Who?

Let us examine how a provider–author can incorporate the Reporter's Formula into his or her patient interviews, analyses, and communication. While it is true that the *who* portion of the formula may be very standard for patient record documentation—who is the patient being discussed?—it is only one of the many ways that answering the question "Who?" can help enhance your documentation. For example, you might want to specify who the patient had been treated by previously, or who accompanied the patient to your office, emergency department (ED), or clinic. Or, as discussed in the revision to the Nurse's Notes in Chapter 3, detailing who, in terms of another provider(s), was also involved in a procedure or patient event can be very beneficial to the reader's interpretation of the record and to the provider–author's credibility.

Think of another question that might be important to answer in your patient record.

_____

_____

_____

What?

The next Reporter's Formula question to consider is *what*. This simple question has a multitude of roles in healthcare providers' interactions, decision making, tests, and outcomes. As you likely have already surmised, there are a breadth of circumstances and contexts in which a provider–author would need to obtain answers to the "what" questions, as well as to discuss "what" responses in her or his patient record. For example, here are a few "what" questions that should be considered by providers–authors depending on the patient, the circumstances, and the document to be created:

- What happened?
- What were you doing at the time you noticed _____?
- What medicines do you currently take?
- What are you allergic to?
- What can I help you with today?
- What do you remember about the event?
- What happened the last time this occurred?
- What were your results previously?
- What was the reason I (provider) did _____?
- What caused me (provider) to make that decision or recommendation?
- What specific findings resulted in the treatment plan?
- What were the outcomes of the action–plan?

As you can see, "what" questions are extremely diverse and very important to your information gathering but also to your analysis of the data that your audience needs and expects. Almost every type of patient record will benefit from a provider–author taking the time to ensure that as many "what" questions as possible, from both a patient's and provider's perspectives, have been asked and answered in the document.

> How do you incorporate "what" responses, from the patient or your self-assessment, into your patient records?
>
> _____
>
> _____
>
> _____
>
> _____

Where?

Like most of the Reporter's Formula questions, *where* is likely a part of your current data gathering or interviewing process. However, many providers–authors think of the Reporter's Formula questions as helpful in their patient discussions, but not as tools for content analysis of their patient records. Our discussion of this formula is to highlight the value of the formula questions for both your patient communication and information generation but, equally important, for you in analyzing how your documentation addresses the reader's questions and needs. The more you can ingrain the notion that your need for specific answers to questions are likely the same as your audience's needs, the more effective your patient records will become. Therefore, you can use the Reporter's Formula not just to obtain data but to evaluate your communication of that data in your document.

The "where" questions from the Reporter's Formula have many important possibilities based on your patient, the context, document, and issue being discussed. For example, a few of the possible "where" questions for your patients and/or your patient records include the following:

- Where does it hurt?
- Where does the pain go?
- Where were you when you first noticed it?
- Where have you gone to try to find a treatment?
- Where did I (provider) refer the patient?
- Where was I (provider) when I examined or treated the patient?

As you can see, the Reporter's Formula quickly provides you with six possible questions to answer from both content and analysis purposes.

How might the answers to "where" questions help you improve the effectiveness of your communication in a patient record?

_____

_____

_____

When?

Some of the Reporter's Formula can provide redundant information, but if used appropriately, they should help to reinforce or expand upon other answers. The issue of *when* is very important to healthcare providers and their documentation. Readers want to know a number of key answers related to this particular Reporter's Formula question:

- When did you first notice _____?
- When was the last time you _____?
- When were you exposed, treated, or _____?
- When did I (provider) first see the patient?
- When did I (provider) last see the patient?
- When did the patient start the treatment _____?

Clearly, there are many other "when" questions, but our goal here is to highlight a few ways you can use "when" for interviewing patients, data gathering, and analyzing the records you author.

> Think of a patient record you might author in your profession. How would assessing the answers to potential "when" questions in the document help to enhance it from both provider–author and audience perspectives?
>
> _____
>
> _____
>
> _____
>
> _____

Why?

Of all the Reporter's Formula questions, _why_ might be the one question that applies more to your document than to your patient interaction? Certainly, there are times when you will want to ask your patient "why"; however, there are likely many more opportunities to use "why" analysis in your assessment of the communication effectiveness of your patient record and what it communicates about why you did certain exams, tests, and treatments. But also, why you did not do others. Some examples of when you might use "why" include the following:

- Why did you choose today to seek treatment?
- Why did you not take the medicine as prescribed?
- Why did you decide not to follow the plan we agreed upon?
- Why did I (provider) order those tests?
- Why did I not (provider) do _____?
- Why did I (provider) recommend that treatment, plan, or action?

> Think of a patient record you might author in your profession. How would assessing your answers to potential "why" questions in the document help to enhance it from both provider–author and audience perspectives?
>
> _____
>
> _____
>
> _____
>
> _____

How?

One of the most important Reporter's Formula questions is *how*. Readers need to know how an injury occurred. They also want to know how the patient's illness or injury was evaluated and treated. Answers to "how" questions apply to numerous aspects of your patient interactions, treatment plans, and course of care. Some examples of when you might use "how" in your discussions and documentations include the following:

- How did this happen?
- How did you respond to the medicine or treatment?
- How did you treat this when it happened before?
- How is the treatment plan working?
- How do I intend to discuss the possible treatment choices with the patient and/or family?

> Think of a patient record you might author in your profession. Evaluate the ways "how" questions might help you create more effective patient documents from both provider–author and audience perspectives?
>
> _____
> _____
> _____
> _____

Your ability to effectively incorporate the Reporter's Formula into your patient interviews, data gathering, and into your pre-authoring and re-authoring processes will be rewarded with enhanced information exchange with patients and analyses of what information your audience expects and what your document communicates.

REFERENCE

Abbott, B., & Costello, L. (2000). *Who's on First?* Retrieved on February 19, 2009, from http://www.baseball-almanac.com/humor4.shtml.

Chapter 5

Using the Authoring Process

Making It Work

Everyone in health care today understands the time constraints, pressures, and demands of patient care. Regardless of your role (MD, DO, APRN, PA, RN, PT), the old maxim—there are only two certainties in life, death and taxes—has evolved to three certainties: death, taxes, and too little time. However, as you will see in Chapter 7, time constraints will not be an effective legal defense if your patient records are unclear and/or do not fulfill their intended purposes. Nor will it be acceptable to your colleagues, supervisors, and the administration if the records do not communicate effectively for their intended readers (Nursing Link, 2009; Pagano & Jacocks, 1992; Pagano & Ragan, 1992; Szauter, Ainsworth, Holden, & Mercado, 2006). Therefore, one of the goals of this text is not just to help you enhance your written communication effectiveness but also to learn a process that does not further impact your time constraints.

It would seem logical to assume that at this point you are rolling your eyes, shaking your head, or performing some other nonverbal behavior that illustrates your skepticism and/or disbelief. And if you have graduated from a professional school and have been working in health care, you may even be using verbal messages to communicate your distrust. However, I am here to assure you that this is not a hoax or a falsehood. The reality is that learning how to author patient records using this process requires skills that have to be assimilated, practiced, and refined. But once you learn these skills, you will be able to adapt and adjust them as needed for each patient record and its intended audience, purpose, and use.

The Record

Because the patient records you are required to author are particular to your profession, this book will discuss these documents both generically and individually. The important thing to understand is that the use of the authoring process we have discussed is the same for each patient record you will need to create (for example, History and Physical, Nurse's Notes, Reports, Discharge Summary, and so forth). So, let us get started on practicing the process and honing the skill.

> When you first start playing a video game, do you get beyond level 2 or 3 the first time? If no, why not? If yes, please tell me how you do it.
>
> _____
>
> _____
>
> _____

Throughout our lives, we are constantly learning, practicing, and improving various skills. Think about a baby who first learns to form sounds, then words, then sentences, and so on. If you learned to play a musical instrument, you had to start out slowly mastering the keys and notes. Authoring patient records is no different. The problem is that you already have mastered the skill of authoring other types of documents, such as letters, e-mails, and research papers. Therefore, it seems almost intuitive that if you know how to author one form of written communication, it should be no problem to author patient records. But let us explore that thinking for just a minute. You have been walking all your life, so do you think you can step onto a dance floor and be an effective dancer? Think of the years of practice and training it takes a ballerina to become an expert (the same feet and legs that she uses every day for walking, climbing, or running). Or, how about when you advanced from riding a bike to driving a car; it involved the same principle—getting you from here to there but using totally different skills, and therefore, it took a while for you to master the clutch, brakes, and steering. Or, what about the skill that makes so many people insane: trying to learn to hit a stationary golf ball the direction you intend?

The point of this discussion is that skills require assimilation and practice. If you can accept that reality, then you can improve your authoring of patient records. Let us begin by discussing how we are going to put into practice the process we discussed previously. We can begin by creating a checklist for initially using the process:

1. Understand what is expected for each patient record you may need to author.
2. Learn the authoring process.
3. Practice the skill.
4. Get feedback.
5. Revise the document.
6. Get feedback.
7. Revise the document if needed.
8. Proofread.
9. Revise as needed.
10. Sign the document.

One of the reasons to begin with a simple checklist is that it clearly illustrates the iterative process that effective healthcare providers–authors need to master.

What Is Expected?

Regardless of your profession or role, each patient record you author has certain preconceived expectations by potential users of that document. As we have discussed previously, you need to fully understand your audience's needs–expectations. For example, if you are creating a History & Physical (H&P), you should recognize that most readers will expect the author and, therefore, the document to communicate at a minimum the following patient information:

- Name, age, sex, race, and vital signs
- Chief complaint (as a quote from the patient if possible)
- Present history (details of the current illness, problem, or injury; including all reported symptoms and any signs, e.g., temperature at home, blood pressure from home health provider, etc.)
- Past history (diagnosed medical conditions, surgeries, trauma–injuries, hospitalizations, and pregnancies; current prescriptions; allergies to medicines or food)
- Family history (major illnesses of grandparents, parents, and siblings; including hereditary conditions such as cardiovascular diseases, diabetes, kidney diseases, cancer, etc.)
- Social history (including tobacco [packs, cigars, chews per day]; alcohol [beer, wine, or liquor cans/glasses per week]; and/or drug use; marital status; sexual history [i.e., number of sexual contacts, sexually transmitted diseases (STDs), birth control, condom use]; career–work status)
- Review of systems
- Physical examination
- Test results (lab, x-ray, EKG, etc.)
- Assessment or working diagnosis
- Initial treatment plan

Therefore, an author of an H&P can quickly review this list and ensure she or he has obtained the information from the patient–family, examination, and any test results needed to address each of these expected sections of an H&P. Clearly, as part of your professional and clinical education, you learned, or will be learning, how to gather the information needed for each of these sections and how to assimilate that data and use critical thinking to arrive at a working diagnosis and initial treatment plan. Consequently, the information you obtain will be a collection of subjective data (what the patient feels or thinks), historical data (what the patient recalls or was told), and objective data (what your examination findings and tests include).

It is this amalgamation of information that readers expect and an author needs to address in his or her H&P. The quantity of information supplied for each of these sections is up to the author and should be determined by the patient's illness or injury and the reason for creating the document as well as the purpose and use for it.

Will there be any difference in the quantity of information your readers might expect if you are authoring an H&P for a 75-year-old patient who is being admitted to the Medical Intensive Care Unit (MICU) with a cerebrovascular accident (CVA) versus a pre-employment H&P for a healthy 30-year-old? If so, why? If no, why not?

Part of the issue for authors of patient records is how much information to supply in a particular patient's record. The goal of this text is to help you understand that you need to supply whatever quantity and detail of information an intended audience needs to know. This documented information should basically be the same as what the provider needs to make decisions about the patient's illness or injury, treatment, complications, and so forth. A good way to help you determine the quantity of data to provide assessment is to return to our earlier discussion of replication. As was mentioned, if you want your readers to be able to use your document to replicate what you heard and observed and use that data to arrive at the same conclusion as you, then you need to supply all of the information necessary to accomplish that goal. However, when in doubt, it is always better to supply more information than too little.

Learning the Authoring Process

This book is intended to assist you in learning the authoring process by helping you understand how the pre-authoring, authoring, re-authoring, and proofreading functions enhance your written communication, goal attainment, and desired outcome. For whatever document you need to create, you first should quickly assess what data you and, therefore, readers need to evaluate the patient context (annual physical, post-op status, acute trauma, and so forth) being discussed. Then, you need to use the Reporter's Formula plus your interviewing and physical examination skills to collect information from the patient or family members, test results, physical findings, and so on. That is all part of your pre-authoring. Once you have gathered that information, you need to analyze how much of the data need to be communicated to accomplish your record's intended purpose(s).

> How do you differentiate between subjective and objective data? And, what is the difference between signs and symptoms?
>
> _____
>
> _____
>
> _____
>
> _____

For example, if you needed to author a report using a Subjective, Objective, Assessment, Plan (SOAP) Note for a 33-year-old, African American, male carpenter who has a closed fracture of his left thumb, your pre-authoring process would include the following:

1. What information do you and your readers need to know about the patient's injury, present and past history?
   a. Use the Reporter's Formula to gather it.
2. What details from your physical exam are needed?
3. What is your working diagnosis–assessment?
4. What is your treatment plan, and why, if needed?

Your interview, Reporter's Formula, exam, and tests generated the following information:

- On 2/2/2002, a metal toolbox fell off a shelf at work and landed on the patient's left hand, and he came directly from work to your Occupational Health Clinic.

- He is on no daily medications, has no allergies, and has no chronic illnesses.
- Vital signs: pulse = 90; respiration = 14; blood pressure = 148/92.
- Left hand = edema over posterior left hand with hematoma of left thumb from metacarpal-phalangeal (MCP) joint to tuft. No laceration. No subungual hematoma. Full range of motion (ROM) all digits of left hand without pain, except in left thumb. Full extension left thumb with pain, unable to flex left thumb at proximal-interphalangeal joint (PIP) beyond 45 degrees due to pain. Sensation intact in all digits of left hand. Snuff box nontender.
- X-ray of left hand = nondisplaced fracture, proximal phalanx left thumb.

A SOAP Note is a type of report that can be used by almost any provider–author in a wide variety of settings (hospital, clinic, home health, and so forth). A SOAP Note includes the following:

Subjective information from the patient or family about an illness, injury, course of treatment, or problem.

Objective data gathered by a health provider (vital signs, examination, tests, procedures, treatments, etc.).

Assessment is the provider–author's analysis of the subjective and objective findings.

Plan is the provider's intended course of action, hopefully based on a patient-centered approach that includes the patient and/or family members in the decision-making process.

Skills Application

1. Which data above do you think must be included in your SOAP Note for this patient, and why?

_____

_____

_____

_____

_____

_____

_____

2. Who are included in the primary audience for this SOAP Note?

   _____

   _____

   _____

3. How does the fact that the patient was injured at work impact your pre-authoring decisions about the information to include in this SOAP Note? Why?

   _____

   _____

   _____

   _____

4. Use the pre-authoring data you identified in Question Nos. 1, 2, and 3 above to create a SOAP Note for this patient.

   S_____

   _____

   _____

   O_____

   _____

   _____

   A_____

   _____

   _____

   P_____

   _____

   _____

This exercise was intended to help you better understand how to use pre-authoring data gathering and analyses to inform your authoring of a patient record. As we discussed earlier in this chapter, the authoring process is iterative, so once you have something on paper (in this case), dictated, or on a computer, you can review it based on your pre-authoring analyses compared to what you actually communicated in the document. This back and forth (between the pre-authoring assessment and the actual messages documented) provides self-feedback for you as an author. In an ideal situation, an author would benefit from asking a member of the potential audience (professor, colleague, team member, and so forth) to read the document and offer an assessment from a reader's perspective. While this is an excellent way for healthcare providers–authors to get feedback on their documents, it is frequently impossible from a time and/or personnel perspective. Therefore, having a quasi-objective method for self-assessing the message you created is invaluable. Early in your assimilation and practice of the authoring process, you will want to actually jot down your pre-authoring analyses. However, as you become more practiced and skilled, you will be able to do pre-authoring without the need for notes, and you will be able to quickly compare your actual document to your mental pre-authoring analyses for feedback and any needed revisions. Let us look at an example of what the pre-authoring for the patient above might have generated.

1. What data do you think must be included in your SOAP Note for this patient and why?

   Because this is a workers' compensation patient (injured at work), the purpose for this document is a bit different than it would be if the patient was not injured at work. Consequently, the SOAP Note needs to include the who, what, when, where, why, and how related to the injury. As with other types of reports, the patient's significant past medical history, including current medications and allergies, will be necessary to record. Besides the vital signs, the physical examination of the patient's hand, especially ROM, sensation, and any lacerations or puncture wounds, will be important to communicate to readers. The patient's x-ray findings and treatment plan, including work status, will also be critical. Finally, while it is not directly related to his workers' compensation office visit, it will be important to discuss the patient's elevated blood pressure since he denies a history of chronic illnesses.

   Remember the amount of detail in a SOAP Note (regardless of whether it is for a clinic, hospital, or home visit) is context-dependent. So, a SOAP Note for a routine follow-up office visit may be very brief and still supply the information needed by an audience. This may be very different from the detail needed in a SOAP Note for a new injury seen in the same office. The provider has to determine how much information readers and, consequently the SOAP Note, require based on the reason for the patient's visit, the findings, assessment, and plan.

2. Who are included in the primary audience for this SOAP Note?

   The primary audience for this SOAP Note would include other healthcare providers who might care for the patient, including the patient's primary care provider (PCP). In addition, because this is a workers' compensation case, the patient's employer and the workers' compensation company as well as the state workers' compensation commission–board are all potential primary readers of this document.

3. How does the fact that the patient was injured at work impact your pre-authoring decisions about the information to include in this SOAP Note? Why?

    Because this is a workers' compensation case, the employer will want to know, besides the diagnosis, what is the patient's work status: regular duty, modified duty, or out of work. And, the worker's compensation company who will be paying for the services rendered will want to know the specifics about the events that led to the injury, the specifics about the events and the physical examination (if there is any question about the where or when the injury occurred and your record of the patient's communication may be compared to what the patient told the employer), and any specialist referrals. Therefore, much more detail about the events surrounding the injury will be more important to your primary audience than they would be if, for example, the patient tripped over his dog and fractured his finger at home.

How does this pre-authoring analysis compare with the one you completed? In the present example, the impact of the patient being injured at work is very significant for your pre-authoring analyses. The quantity and specifics of the information needed for a SOAP Note about a work-related injury are very different from the same Note for a nonwork-related injury or illness. Similarly, the patient's elevated blood pressure, which may be related to his pain but could be due to prehypertension and pain or undiagnosed hypertension, is important to document, even though it has little or no relevance to the work-related injury you are treating. In addition, while the workers' compensation insurance company and the patient's employer, two of your primary audiences for this document, may not be interested in his blood pressure, other health-care providers will be, and that audience will want to know that the author recognized the potential problem, analyzed it, and took appropriate steps to educate the patient about it and have it further evaluated. Based on this pre-authoring analysis, let us examine how these actions could be used to author the patient's SOAP Note.

SOAP Note

S. 2/2/2002, 33 y/o B   c/o pain in his L. thumb. Patient states that he is a carpenter who was at work today when his metal toolbox fell off a shelf onto his L. posterior hand. He came directly from work to this office. He denies any chronic medical illnesses or previous injury to his L. thumb. He takes no daily medications and has no known drug allergies.

O. VS: P. 90, R. 14, BP. 148/92, L. hand is edematous over post. metacarpals and L. thumb. No lac., abrasion, or puncture wounds. Full ROM in all digits except L. thumb. Sensation intact in distal tuft of all L. hand digits, including thumb. Hematoma, L. thumb from MCP to distal tuft, no subungual hematoma. Flexion L. thumb to 45° with pain in PIP joint, full extension with pain at PIP joint. No snuff-box tenderness or pain with ROM. X-ray L. hand shows nondisplaced fx L. thumb proximal phalanx.

A. 1. Nondisplaced fracture L. thumb. 2. Contusion L. hand.

P. Padded, aluminum splint in position of function L. thumb. Ice for 24–36 hours as frequently as possible to L. hand and thumb. Ibuprofen 800 mg. now, then q 8 hours with food prn pain or swelling. Elevate thumb to decrease pain. Recheck in 1 week. Return to work on light duty with no use of left hand for gripping, lifting, pushing, or pulling.

We have now taken our pre-authoring patient information and our audience and document analyses and used them to author this SOAP Note. We could stop there, sign it, and make it a legal document, or we could review it quickly to see if there are any major content problems or miscommunication. But, just reading over something you have recently authored is frequently not very helpful because your mind may fill in missing words or read sentences the way you intended to author them instead of how they are actually documented. So, it helps to have an outside reader, or a checklist of some kind—either written down or in your head—to examine against what you authored.

If we look at the pre-authoring exercise we did, we can compare it to the document and give ourselves some feedback about whether or not we accomplished the goals we established and presented the material we felt was important to meet the primary readers' needs and expectations as well as the purpose for the document. Therefore, comparing the pre-authoring analysis of the data that needs to be communicated in this SOAP Note, with the audience, purpose, and use assessments, we can see that the record is clearly written for healthcare providers and for the patient's employer and workers' compensation insurance company. The SOAP Note documents the who, what, when, where, and how of this injury. In addition, the record details the physical examination and x-ray findings, along with the provider–author's assessment and treatment plan, including work status. However, upon evaluation, we can see that the current SOAP Note does not do something that was identified in pre-authoring as important, and that is a discussion of the patient's elevated blood pressure and a follow-up with the patient's primary care provider (PCP). Consequently, now that we have used our pre-authoring to provide feedback on what was authored, we can quickly go back and re-author the document.

SOAP Note (Revised)

S. 2/2/2002, 33 y/o B   c/o pain in his L. thumb. Patient states that he is a carpenter who was at work today when his metal toolbox fell off a shelf onto his L. posterior hand. He came directly from work to this office. He denies any chronic medical illnesses or previous injury to his L. thumb. He takes no daily medications and has no known drug allergies.

O. VS: P. 90, R. 14, BP. 148/92, L. hand is edematous over post. metacarpals and L. thumb. No lac., abrasion, or puncture wounds. Full ROM in all digits except L. thumb. Sensation intact in distal tuft of all L. hand digits, including thumb. Hematoma, L. thumb from MCP to distal tuft, no subungual hematoma. Flexion L. thumb to 45° with pain in PIP joint, full extension with pain at PIP joint. No snuff-box tenderness or pain with ROM. X-ray L. hand shows nondisplaced fx L. thumb proximal phalanx.

A. 1. Nondisplaced fracture L. thumb. 2. Contusion L. hand.

3. Blood Pressure Elevation—etiology undetermined, pain, prehypertension and pain, or undiagnosed hypertension must be ruled out.

P. Padded, aluminum splint in position of function L. thumb. Ice for 24–36 hours as frequently as possible to L. hand and thumb. Ibuprofen 800 mg. now, then q 8 hours with food prn pain or swelling. Elevate thumb to decrease pain. Recheck in 1 week. Return to work on light duty with no use of left hand for gripping, lifting, pushing, or pulling. Follow-up with PCP regarding BP recheck and further evaluation ASAP.

We have used our feedback from our review of the pre-authoring analyses against the completed document to revise the SOAP Note to meet our goals and to better achieve our intended outcome—effective written communication that meets the readers' needs and expectations and the document's intended purpose and use (see highlighted revised areas). But one last step remains before we are ready to sign this document and make it a legal patient record. We need to read through it to ensure that there are no misspelled or missing words or typos. Once we have completed proofreading the document, it is ready to be signed (in pen or electronically).

This iterative process of analyzing the contents needed, the audience and their expectations, and the document's intended purpose and use and comparing that data against the information communicated in the completed record is the benefit of using the authoring process. This process affords healthcare providers an opportunity not only to analyze the audience, purpose, use, and necessary content for creating any patient record prior to authoring it but to use that analysis to evaluate the authored record and revise as needed to make it communicate more effectively.

REFERENCES

Nursing Link. (2009). *Medical record keeping for health care providers*. Retrieved on February 25, 2009, from http://www.nursinglink.com/training/articles/352-medical-record-keeping-for-health-care-providers.

Pagano, M., & Jacocks, M. (1992). *Communicating effectively in medical records: A guide for physicians*. Newbury Park, CA: Sage.

Pagano, M., & Ragan, S. (1992). *Communication skills for professional nurses*. Newbury Park, CA: Sage.

Szauter, K., Ainsworth, M., Holden, M., & Mercado, A. (2006). Do students do what they write and write what they do? The match between the patient encounter and patient note. *Academic Medicine, 81*(10), S44–S47.

Chapter 6

Written, Dictated, and Electronic Patient Records

The Format Issue

This chapter will help you explore the major formats for patient records: handwritten, dictated and transcribed, or computerized. As you know, more and more organizations are moving toward electronic patient records. However, these efforts have been slowed by a number of major issues that will be discussed later in this chapter. Therefore, in lieu of a total conversion to an electronic format, patient records continue to be authored as handwritten narratives, reports, and checklists, or as dictated and transcribed documents. Let us examine the differences for both the provider–author and the intended audience for each of these formats.

> If you have to communicate a message (nonface to face) to someone about something, what is your favorite format (phone–verbal, electronic [IM, text, or e-mail], or handwritten)? Why?

Handwritten Records

As Benjamin Franklin (1754) first reported (see Chapter 1), for over 250 years patient documentation in this country has been required and created predominantly in handwritten records. These handwritten documents have a number of positive aspects for the provider–author:

- There is no need for electronic equipment.
- They only require a pen and paper.
- They can be authored anywhere.
- No third party (transcriptionist or computer) is needed.
- They require no equipment training.
- Author is solely responsible for documentation.

While the positive aspects for providers–authors are numerous, there are negative issues related to handwritten patient records as well:

- Organization and order of content is determined by the author.
- Breadth and depth of content is up to the author.
- Ease of documentation can lead to procrastination.
- There is no forced delay between authoring, proofreading, and signing.

As you think about authoring patient records, you will likely be influenced by a number of factors, including your age, experience in health care, and computer skills. However, in spite of those personal concerns, there are a number of common attributes and deficiencies that we should explore.

Handwritten patient records allow providers–authors to document information quickly and easily. They require few additional tools (a pen and paper), and they can be authored at the bedside, in an office, or at the nurse's station. Handwritten records do not require any special skills (typing, computing, or dictating), nor do they necessitate any additional equipment or personnel (transcriptionists, IT, telephone software, dictation machine, computers, computer software, and so forth). However, from a provider–author perspective, handwritten documents do have some shortcomings.

First, we need to point out that there are two basic types of handwritten records: narrative and checklists. A narrative-type document is one where the provider–author determines what information, in what order, and in what quantity it will be supplied. These would include Subjective, Objective, Assessment, Plan (SOAP) Notes, or other template-type (nonchecklist) records, that provide a structure for the document in which the provider–author determines how much information to communicate. Conversely, a checklist typically provides little or no area for an extended narrative discussion(s) of various findings. Instead, the checklist format forces a provider–author to address–answer a prescribed set of statements, questions, or topics related to the patient's interview, exam, test, or treatment.

For nonchecklist, handwritten records, the provider–author has to determine the organization and order of the message (SOAP, unstructured narrative, subheadings, and so forth). In addition, each provider–author must assess the breadth and depth of the content communicated to meet the primary and secondary audiences' needs. Even with checklist, handwritten records, providers–authors have to determine if the amount of information communicated with mere check marks is sufficient to fulfill the purpose for the document and the readers' expectations.

Another concern for providers–authors of patient records is related to the ease of documentation. Because a handwritten record can be created any time, many authors procrastinate and do not author their records until hours, days, weeks, or even months after the interaction, exam, or procedure. While this procrastination creates memory issues for the provider–author, it also causes financial problems for the institution because the patient's insurance frequently cannot be billed until the record is completed.

Just as troubling for providers–authors who create their records in a timely fashion is the reality that handwritten documents are expected to be signed at the time they are written. In previous chapters, we discussed the valuable role proofreading plays in the authoring process; however, proofreading works best when an author can put some time between authoring and proofreading. With handwritten records, there is little, if any, time between these two phases of the authoring process. Consequently, it is not uncommon to find missing words, misspelled words, or unclear sentences in signed, handwritten records. These pros and cons for handwritten patient records apply to providers–authors, but the realities of this format have even broader implications for readers' of handwritten documents.

What do you think are two of the key problems for readers of handwritten patient records?

As you may know, readers have a number of problems with handwritten patient records. First and foremost, however, readers frequently have difficulty reading provider–authors' handwriting. This is a major problem since healthcare providers' readers need to accurately decode their writing in order to fulfill orders, understand treatment plans and decision making, and approve compensation. Another issue for readers related to handwritten patient records is the frequently abbreviated or condensed content that lacks specificity, description, or explanation. It can be argued that this is not related to the format, but instead to a provider–author's communication decisions. However, because of the time required to physically write a patient record, it is not surprising that the quantity of content would be negatively impacted by this format.

Interestingly, checklists can also be faulted for a lack of detail, specificity, and explanation as well. By reducing patient records to a routinized list of topics or statements, readers are limited in the amount of information they can expect to obtain. For example, it is entirely possible to have a checklist that does not include a category or topic that is needed for a particular patient's condition or situation. Let us examine a portion of an Emergency Department (ED) checklist.

Checklist Example

PAST HX

Diabetes: Type 1 _____ Type 2 _____

Hepatitis/HIV _____

Tetanus _____

Meds _____ Aspirin/Coumadin/Clopidogrel

Allergies _____ NKDA _____

SOCIAL HX

Smoker _____ Drugs _____

Alcohol _____ Occupation _____

FAMILY HX

Negative _____ (T-System, 2008)

QUESTIONS

1. Do you find this checklist for the patient's past, social, and family histories helpful? If yes, why? If no, why not?

    _____

    _____

    _____

2. If your patient had a history of angina, heart failure, or even hypertension, how and where would you document it on this checklist?

    _____

    _____

    _____

While checklists can be very helpful to providers–authors in terms of saving time and minimizing legibility issues related to other forms of handwritten records, they also create problems for authors and readers. For example, does the fact that information is not included mean it was obtained but not recorded? Or, does the lack of information mean it was never asked or examined? Does the fact that certain information is not listed on the checklist imply that it is not needed? For example, the checklist sections above are taken from a "Prototype Emergency Physician Record MVC" (T System, 2008, p. 1). If used as documentation for a patient who was involved in a motor vehicle collision–crash (MVC), would a reader not be concerned about the patient's past cardiac or pulmonary history (might it not have contributed to the cause of the collision or be triggered by it)? What about the patient's neurologic or musculoskeletal past history (might it be helpful to know that the patient had a previous fractured pelvis, femur, and so forth)? Would the patient's marital status be an important part of the social history (if nothing else, to know who to contact)?

The point of this discussion is that checklists, by their very nature, are prescribed topic areas and questions or statements to be answered, but if the provider–author merely checks the appropriate lines or boxes (as intended by the format), does that fulfill his or her obligations for a reader? Clearly, the answer to that question will be context-related. For a patient with otitis media, a checklist might be sufficient to document all the information an audience needs to assess the problem and the provider–author's examination, decision making, and treatment plan. However, in more complicated and multisystem impacted patients, is a checklist sufficient to address the primary and secondary audiences' needs and expectations? Do you think 2 or 3 years later the check marks on a checklist will supply you, as the author, with enough data to recall what you learned, saw, did, and why (in case you have to respond to a lawyer's questions in a deposition or court)?

The reality for providers–authors of checklists is awareness—just because something is not on the list does not mean it should be ignored based on the patient, the problem, the context, and the audience, purpose, and use for the document. In some situations, the provider–author may feel it is necessary to include additional data separately; however, with most checklists, there is precious little space to enter any additional information, and there is no assurance that any documentation done on a separate sheet of paper will be stored or scanned with the checklist record. Therefore, this issue of the quantity and specificity of information provided remains a major concern for readers of most handwritten patient records (both checklists and nonchecklists). However, patient records that are handwritten are not the only format that cause problems for providers–authors and/or audiences.

Dictated and Transcribed Records

As you think about the differences between handwritten patient records and dictated and transcribed records, you should immediately recognize some important distinctions:

- Dictated records should not have legibility issues.
- Dictated records take time to get into the patient's chart.
- Dictated records provide a time delay for authors before proofreading.
- Dictated records can create re-authoring issues.

As discussed above, handwritten records are frequently confusing, unclear, or even unable to be read based on the penmanship of the provider–author. Therefore, one distinct potential advantage of transcribed dictation is its legibility. However, a reader's ability to interpret the written symbols on a typed document does not ensure effective communication.

Have you ever typed a paper for a class and had the professor comment that sentences or paragraphs were unclear? If so, why do you think the professor felt they were unclear?

_____

_____

_____

Authoring documents for a class or in a patient's record can be aided by using a format that minimizes penmanship–legibility issues. However, that does not change the need for providers–authors to understand and meet their audience's needs for content, clarity, and explanation. Therefore, merely changing the format for your patient records does not, in and of itself, alleviate a provider–author's need to use the authoring process to communicate clearly and effectively to his or her audience. Let us look at an example.

Pathology Report #1

Preoperative Diagnosis: Abdominal pain.

Operative Findings: (blank on original.)

Specimen Submitted: Gallbladder.

Gross Description: The specimen consists of a gallbladder approximately 7 cm long, which contains a shred of apposed liver tissue. The gallbladder contains numerous firm, yellow, calculi, which vary from 1 mm to 8 mm in diameter. The gallbladder is less than 1 mm in thickness and contains a number of bright yellow streaks focally. Representative tissue is submitted for histology.

Microscopic: Examined by pathologist 11/8/____.

Impression: Acute gangrenous cholecystitis and cholelithiasis.

Comment: There is considerable acute and chronic inflammation in the fat with necrosis adjacent to the gallbladder.

QUESTIONS

1. What is your response as a reader of this document?

2. What are the major purposes for this provider–author (pathologist) to create this patient record?

3. Where in this record does the provider–author describe the microscopic findings of inflammation that is reported in the Impression, "Acute gangrenous cholecystitis . . ."?

Reading Pathology Report #1, a typed, likely transcribed, record of a pathologist's dictation of a specimen removed in the operating room leaves readers with at least one major question. Where are the signs of acute cholecystitis? As a reader of this record, we would expect to know enough information about the specimen to reach the same impression as the pathologist–author; however, even though this is a typed document that has no penmanship or legibility issues for a reader, there are still content problems that the provider–author failed to consider or chose to ignore. If the purpose of a patient report (like Pathology Report #1) was merely for a professional to state his or her impression, then these documents would be much more succinct and just provide a diagnosis or impression. But, that is not the only purpose for these documents. In fact, one of the purposes primary and secondary readers expect to be fulfilled are the specifics of the findings that result in the provider–author's impression. Consequently, the lack of any description of the microscopic changes to the gallbladder in Pathology Report #1 makes readers question, if it was inflamed and gangrenous, why was there not a discussion of the microscopic findings that should demonstrate such changes?

Too often, providers–authors communicate only a portion of the information that readers need to arrive at the same conclusions–impressions as the author. And while it is true that the author of Pathology Report #1 is a specialist, it is also true that the purpose for this document is to communicate her or his findings so the audience can assess the evaluation and replicate (at least intellectually) the provider–author's tests and assessment and determine his or her credibility and the impression's validity.

To see how a different provider–author creates a pathology report, please examine the following.

Pathology Report #2

Specimen: Scalene node.

History: Lymphoma.

Gross: Specimen consists of a yellow, fatty piece of tissue measuring up to 4.0 cm in greatest diameter, which contains a rubbery nodule measuring 1.5 cm in greatest dimension. Representative sections are submitted in two cassettes.

Microscopic: Histologic exam reveals sections of lymph node tissue comprised of expanded nodules composed of neoplastic lymphocytes representing a mixture of small noncleaved and cleaved cells. Moderate numbers of mitoses are identified. There is invasion of the capsule and extension into the adjacent adipose tissue by the lymphocytic elements.

Diagnosis: Non-Hodgkin's lymphoma, follicular-mixed cleaved and noncleaved cell type (550–820G).

QUESTIONS

1. What is your response as a reader of this document?

   _____

   _____

   _____

2. What are the major purposes for this provider–author (pathologist) to create this patient record?

   _____

   _____

   _____

3. Can you as a reader assess the provider–author's diagnosis? Why or why, not? And if so, how?

   _____

   _____

   _____

As you no doubt observed, Pathology Report #2 does not rely on the provider–author's credibility and simple statement of the diagnosis. Instead, the pathologist–author provides detailed microscopic descriptions of the specimen. Consequently, a reader can assess the diagnosis not solely on the author's opinion but on the same data the pathologist used to make his or her assessment. When you compare the Microscopic section of Pathology Reports #1 and #2, you can quickly see a difference in the apparent pre-authoring and re-authoring assessments by the two pathologists. The author of Pathology Report #1 does not appear to value documentation for replication. Pathology Report #1 has no information at all about the microscopic findings, only the fact that the pathologist examined the specimen and the date. However, the author of Pathology Report #2 clearly wants her or his readers to be able to at least virtually replicate the microscopic findings. Therefore, Pathology Report #2 carefully documents what is seen microscopically so the diagnosis makes perfect sense to a reader, and there is no credibility or validity issues for the provider–author of Pathology Report #2.

The point of these two examples is that using a format that eliminates the problems frequently encountered with handwritten documents does not ensure a provider–author a positive outcome. While the format used to create a patient record does have some impact on the audience's ability to use it and on the provider–author's attainment of his or her communication goals, the reality is that authors still need to practice an authoring process that affords them the best opportunity to meet their readers' needs and the record's purpose.

How do you see the act of dictating a patient record as different for a provider–author than handwriting one? Be specific.

_____

_____

_____

Dictating a patient record is in many ways very similar to handwriting without the physical act of writing the document. Therefore, if you are doing a SOAP Note, for example, you would still organize the document by subjective, objective, assessment, and plan; however, you now have to think aloud. Instead of writing the information, you have to tell the transcriptionist every detail. So, when you might have merely written "I feel better" as your subjective finding, in dictation, you would need to be very clear what you are saying and how it should appear in the document. An example of a dictated subjective finding for a patient might sound like this:

Dictation Example #1

Provider–Author: This is a SOAP Note on John Jones, patient number 22222222, seen and dictated on 9/9/09 by (author's name and title). New paragraph, capital S period, start quote, I feel better period, close quote.

This brief example illustrates how a provider–author who is dictating a patient record and who is trying to ensure control over the transcribed document needs to be meticulous in her or his dictation. On the other hand, a different provider–author might dictate the same information with much less specificity.

Dictation Example #2

Provider–Author: (author's name and title) SOAP Note on John Jones, 22222222, 9/9/09, S, I feel better. O. . .

While providers can use such an abbreviated style, the risk is that the transcriptionist will have to make decisions about what is a quote and where and how to punctuate it. If a provider–author wants to minimize miscommunication and redictating or hand correcting a typed document, then the provider–author needs to be very clear and precise in his or her dictation. And, this specificity does not just pertain to the content of the record but includes its organization, grammar, and style. In the case of dictation, the provider–author should understand that the transcriptionist is responsible for capturing the exact dictation but not for revising it or formatting it. The more you as an author dictating a record can recognize the fact that you should be saying aloud everything you would normally be doing if you were handwriting the record, the better it will be for the document, the transcriptionist, the reader and, therefore, for you as the author.

Another issue related to dictated and transcribed patient records is re-authoring and/or proofreading. Generally, it takes hours, or even days, for a dictated record to get transcribed and returned to the provider–author for her or his signature. As we have discussed previously, this delay between authoring, dictating, and signing frequently makes it easier for the provider–author to identify any misstatements, missing information, or typos while proofreading. However, the problem unique to transcribed provider–authored patient records is the issue of re-authoring. Do you make handwritten changes to the typed document (and include your initials and the date that the changes were made)? Or, do you redictate the record? Or, do you dictate an addendum? Each of these choices has their own pros and cons. Clearly, making the changes in handwriting is problematic in that it requires careful penmanship and documentation of the author's changes and the date. Redictating the record has the advantage of a clean document (assuming there are no typos, and so forth, on the newly transcribed document); however, you technically should record the dictation with the new date, not the prior one. Dictating an addendum is one way to show readers the original and the changes on the same document in a legible format. However, it can be confusing to have the reader go through the record with mistakes and then have to read the addendum further down the page, or on another page, to see that you actually caught and corrected the miscues or miscommunication. In reality, redictating and retranscribing, while it takes a bit longer (dictating, transcribing, and the added time for proofreading the new draft), provides readers with the most accurate and credible information. By taking the time to recreate an error-free document, you eliminate the risk of errors (even corrected ones) distracting the readers' attention away from your content and decision making. Therefore, while dictating and transcribing can enhance some aspects of written communication, it can also raise additional concerns and challenges for a provider–author. However, computerized patient record keeping creates its own unique problems and obstacles for providers–authors.

Electronic Patient Records

One of the hottest topics in health care and politics today is the issue of electronic medical records (EMRs), also referred to as electronic health records and/or electronic patient records. In fact, President Barack Obama has declared, "to improve the quality of our health care while lowering its cost, we will make the immediate investments necessary to ensure that, within 5 years, all of America's medical records are computerized" (Childs, Chang, & Grayson, 2009, para. 2). The purpose of this chapter and this text is not to debate the EMR's potential improvements to the quality of health care; however, few, if any, studies can be found that illustrate objective findings to support this hypothesis. While it is true that using an EMR should eliminate legibility and, therefore, potential errors related to the interpretation of handwritten documents, the risks associated with insufficient content, miscommunication, typos, and so forth, are not eliminated by the use of an EMR.

> What other problems can you perceive in the conversion to an EMR? Be specific.
>
> _____
>
> _____
>
> _____

While there can be little doubt that using an EMR will certainly alter health care in many ways, after using an EMR at two different institutions, the author has observed several shared issues related to authorship by healthcare providers.

- Many healthcare providers are not comfortable typing.
- Typing documents, even if it is predominantly a checklist, frequently takes more time than handwriting or dictating a paper record.
- There is little, if any, opportunity to revise the document.
- Many EMR programs do not include spell-checking software.
- EMRs do not ensure any more thorough interviews or exams by providers. In fact, they may contribute to shortening the interactions between providers and patients.
- Provider reluctance to use an EMR has led to some institutions using a hybrid document that includes: handwritten, dictated, and electronic records for the same patient.

As we explore the use of an EMR, it is important to understand that electronic documentation does not in and of itself ensure more effective record keeping from an effective communication perspective. Callen, Alderton, and McIntosh (2008) found that "the results of our study show it is not necessarily the case that electronic discharge summaries are of higher quality as regards accuracy and completeness than handwritten ones . . ." (p. 619). In fact, the EMRs evaluated in this study created problems for both authors and readers, "across all items studied, the electronic summaries contained a higher number of errors and/or omissions than the handwritten ones" (p. 613). Therefore, the argument that is commonly made by politicians and administrators that simply converting to an EMR will improve the quality of care has not been universally supported by the research to date. The authors of this study postulated that

> possible causes for deficiencies [in the EMRs] include: insufficient training; insufficient education of, and thus realisation by, doctors regarding the importance of accurate, complete discharge summaries; inadequate computer literacy; unfamiliarity with creating discharge summaries electronically; inadequate user interaction design; insufficient integration into routine work processes. (p. 619)

Thus, the notion that merely converting to an EMR will improve the quality of health care seems short-sighted and lacks understanding of both the authoring process and the realities of contemporary healthcare delivery. Many providers, especially those over 40 years of age, may not be comfortable using computers or typing. In addition, with the Health Insurance Portability and Accountability Act (HIPAA) requiring protection of patient information, most institutional computer systems have safeguards that require the computer to be unlocked by a provider with a password after a minute or two of nonuse. This seemingly small step, when required 30 or 40 times a day to access patient records, added to the time it takes to locate the patient's specific record and template for documentation can increase the time it takes to electronically author a record. Add to these steps, the time it takes for an author to type, or check off, his or her information, it is not surprising that electronic authoring of a record can take longer than either handwriting or dictating the same document.

Another problem inherent in using an EMR from an authoring process perspective is the immediacy of the record. It is generally less likely that an author will have time to go back to revise and/or proofread the record prior to electronically signing it. The lack of spell-checking software adds to the author's problem because typing issues can create unexpected typos, misspelled words, incorrect words, or abbreviations (mg versus mcg). And, a provider using an EMR, does not ensure that the interactions, examinations, and treatments were thorough, accurate, or effective. In addition, the provider's use of a computer during an interview or examination may cause the patient to think that the provider was distracted and not focusing on the conversation and/or physical examination.

Finally, it should be noted that some institutions that have converted to an EMR have made the provider–authoring process even more complex by mandating a hybrid format. In response to providers' reluctance to convert to documenting electronically, some healthcare organizations now utilize a hybrid record-keeping system. Within this system, some providers (nurses, PT, and so forth) exclusively document electronically, but physicians, PAs, and APRNs use handwritten checklists, handwritten records, or dictated documents. In fact, the author works in one institution where the providers are using all three formats for every patient seen. That is, a handwritten checklist history–interview form, a dictated–transcribed physical examination form, and computerized documentation for orders, medication, discharge–transfer–admission forms, and so on. As you can imagine, the time constraints imposed by these multiple formats increase time-constraints on the provider as well as on the provider–patient interaction. And as a result of this hybrid format, the institution does not have a true EMR, but instead some patient documents that are handwritten, some transcribed, and some electronic. These multiple formats then get merged, via an additional step, into a hybrid EMR as scanned handwritten and dictated components. And scanned, handwritten records are generally even more difficult to read and interpret from a legibility perspective on a computer screen than on paper.

We have explored some of the problems with converting to an EMR, but currently, the number one problem with converting is that EMRs are not portable. To date, institutions are not sharing electronic records because of privacy and proprietary issues. And while the patient's privacy remains a central concern, the fact is that each institution currently developing EMRs are doing so in a relative vacuum, and therefore, the software they are using is not compatible with the electronic programs being instituted in other hospitals and clinics. So, if a patient is seen in an emergency department in one state, it is almost certain that an EMR created in that ED will not be electronically available to the patient's provider in another state, or even in the same city.

Again, these problems with authoring an EMR are not the focus of this chapter, but it is important for a provider–author to understand the current situation. However, it appears that politicians and administrators are going to continue to drive the evolution to an EMR throughout health care, and therefore, it is imperative for all providers to understand how they differ from an authoring process perspective and how to make them as efficient and as effective a communication tool as possible.

Step one in authoring an EMR versus a handwritten or dictated patient record is to assess the format of the electronic document.

- Is it a stand-alone checklist?
- Does it provide an opportunity for the author to include a narrative?
- How do you sign the document electronically, and at what step in the process is that required?
- Are changes to your record tracked?
- How can the document be amended, if needed, at a later time?
- Is there a way to document unusual or unexpected events apart from the normal template?

Just because you are using an EMR does not eliminate or negate the provider–author's requirement to meet the primary and secondary readers' information needs and expectations for the document. Therefore, if a Nurse's Note, Discharge Summary, PT Report, and so forth, do not provide an expeditious way to document something you as the author feel is important to your patient's health and to the readers' analysis of that patient's care, then you need to find a way to communicate it in the record. Your goal and obligation as a provider–author is to meet the information needs of your primary and secondary readers, regardless of the format of the patient record. It will likely provide little solace to a provider–author who is called before a professional review board or into a courtroom to state that the EMR did not have a box to check or a blank spot for the communication of omitted material–problems.

Let us look at an example of an EMR–Nurse's Note for an ED patient (*Note:* blank space = no information in record; underlined ____ = confidential information redacted).

EMR–Nurse's Note

Date: 02/07/09–1827   **Acct No:** _____

User: _____, RN   **Unit No:** _____

Patient: _____   **Age/Sex:** 43/M

ED Provider: Urgent Care, Dr. _____

Patient Information

Address: _____

Insurance: _____

Next of Kin: _____   **PCP:** No primary care physician

Relation: 01 SPOUSE   **Family Doctor:** _____

Phone: _____

General Data

ED Physician: Urgent Care, Dr. _____   **Arrival Date/Time:** 02/07/09–1740

Practitioner: _____   **Triage Date/Time:** 02/07/09–1806

Nurse: _____

Stated Complaint: Cough, cold, chills

Chief Complaint: Cough   **Priority/Severity:** /9

Allergies

No known drug allergies.

Assessments

02/07/09 1804 Pain Assessment   _____, RN

Scale Used: Number

Intensity: 0

Person Reporting Pain: Patient

02/07/09 1805 Respiratory Assessment   _____, RN

Rate: 20

Effort: Nonlabored

Pattern: Regular

Behavior/LOC: Awake, oriented, cooperative

Cough Description: Nonproductive, harsh, observed

Cough Frequency: Occasional

02/07/09 1806 Triage Form   _____, RN

Verbal or implied consent given for treatment? Y

Triage Note: REPORTS 2 WEEK HX OF INTERMITTENT COUGH AND SINUS CONGESTION NOW WITH 2 DAY HX OF WORSENING COUGH AND CHILLS

Patient's Past Medical History: NA/None

Glasgow Coma Score: 15

Has patient been on isolation in the past? N

Age Appropriate Behavior/Response: Y

Do you feel safe at home? Y

High Nutrition Risk Dx/Condition: None

Learning Barriers: None

Is this patient a fall risk? N

Medications

Prescription/Hx Medication	Type	Issued	Provider	Entered
Polymyxin/Trimethoprim (Polytrim) 10 ML SOLN	Rx	12/07/07	_____	12/07/07
2 DROP OU Q4H, #10 SOLN REF 0				
Guaifenesin/Codeine (Robitussin AC) 5 ML SYRP	Rx	02/07/09	_____	02/07/09

Notes

Entered by _____, RN on 02/07/09 at 1825

Discharged home with instructions and script reviewed and understood

Vital Signs—Adult

Time	Systolic	Diastolic	Pulse Oximetry	Temperature (Fahrenheit)	User
1800	120	75	98	99.4	_____

Time	Respiratory Rate	User
1800	18	_____

QUESTIONS

1. As a secondary reader, what is your overall assessment of the communication effectiveness of this ED EMR?

    _____

    _____

    _____

2. What questions does this EMR create/leave unanswered for readers?

    _____

    _____

    _____

    _____

    _____

3. How do you interpret the lack of a response to the "Priority/Severity/9" score?

    _____

    _____

    _____

While readers of this ED EMR Nurse's Note can agree that it is easy to read from a legibility perspective, it still causes a number of problems for primary and secondary readers. Some of these issues relate to the organization of the document (not likely under the control of the nurse–author), and some of the problems are related to the author's choices for content discussion. For example, the nurse–author informs readers that the patient's chief complaint is a cough; however, in at least two places, the document refers to chills, which are an important consideration. However, there is no mention of recent fevers, the last dose of an antipyretic medication, or any other current medication (only a prescription from an ED visit in 2007). So, readers have no way to assess the complaint of chills and their relationship to any previous temperature elevations.

And while the author likely has no control over the information requested based on the chief complaint, it would seem that readers would appreciate more information related to the present illness. And while it is important to note that this 43-year-old male has no nutrition risks and feels safe at home, it would be equally important to know if he has had any flu-like symptoms, or if his sinus congestion is producing sinus pressure, recent headaches, or a yellow or green nasal discharge. And the lack of data for the "Priority/Severity" calls into question the nurse–author's assessment.

Finally, from an organization of information perspective, this document seems very disorganized with the vital signs at the very end. A statement about the patient's prescription and instructions were given, but we do not know what the diagnosis or assessment of the patient's complaint was, so readers have no way to evaluate the nurse's discharge communication. And there is no mention of what the patient is to do if his symptoms worsen (which is important since the record states he has no PCP and no family doctor). In short, the brevity of information makes this document difficult to use and would likely be impossible to rely on as support for the MD, DO, PA–APRN portion of the EMR.

It would have taken only a sentence or two in the Triage section to discuss the specifics about the patient's chills, for example, "No history of fever and no acetaminophen or ibuprofen in the last 8 hours. No sinus pain, pressure, or nasal discharge reported." And a simple statement in the last Notes section, for example, "Discharged home with upper respiratory instructions that were discussed with the patient who understood. Placed on a single cough medicine prescription and advised to return if symptoms worsen." This approach requires a few extra words, but the difference for the reader is that it is clear what the patient was being treated for, what instructions were provided, and what he should do if he feels worse. It takes very little time to provide more information and clarity for readers; however, it requires a provider–author to analyze what the reader needs and then to supply it.

The important thing for providers–authors of EMRs to remember is the value of using an authoring process that includes audience analysis, pre-authoring, re-authoring, and proofreading. Just because the format changes, it should not result in a change in the authoring process. Effective communication in handwritten, dictated, and/or electronic documents relies on thoughtful and critical analyses by a provider–author. The results will pay enormous dividends for the provider–author, readers, and ultimately, the patient.

E-mail, Websites, and Social Networking

It is impossible to discuss electronic records without also adding e-mail, provider's corporate or personal websites. and social networking (Facebook, MySpace, Twitter, and so forth). Let us begin by considering patient-related e-mails. Many healthcare providers use e-mail to communicate with their colleagues and patients about patient-related health matters. While this is an effective way to rapidly transfer information, it is not without its potential problems and concerns. The legal issues related to e-mail communication will be discussed in Chapter 7; however, it is also important for providers–authors to recognize the pros and cons of this communication channel for patient care.

Pros of Patient-Related E-mails

1. Easy to use.
2. Able to send general information to a large audience with one message.
3. Avoids "telephone tag" (repeatedly leaving voice-mail messages to return call).
4. Provides opportunity to maintain and build a relationship with the patient.
5. Facilitates rapid communication of nonsensitive patient results (lab tests, x-rays, etc.).
6. Offers an opportunity to encourage patients to comply with mutually agreed upon therapy decisions (medications, diet, exercise, etc.).
7. Allows reminders for follow-up visits, scheduled tests, and so forth, without phone calls and voice messages.
8. Delivers an effective method for communicating patient information with consultants and colleagues who are involved in the treatment or care of a common patient.
9. Saves money versus regular mail.
10. Reduces staff time: phoning and mailing.

There are a number of unique opportunities that patient-related e-mail communication presents to healthcare providers. For the most part, it is easy to use, and with a database of patients, providers–authors can use the bcc (blind carbon copy) feature to send a global message to all patients without any of the patients seeing anyone else's e-mail address. E-mail also avoids the all too often problem of a provider returning a patient's call and getting his or her voice mail and then having the patient call back and the provider being unavailable. Even if the message cannot be left in the e-mail, it does afford an opportunity for the provider and patient to negotiate a specific time, date, and phone number to use, or it could recommend the patient call for an appointment to discuss the results of tests. Providers seek to build relationships with patients to maintain their loyalty, to build credibility, and to demonstrate professionalism. E-mail communication is one mechanism for maintaining or building a provider–patient relationship. It is much faster than regular mail, costs nothing per message, and frequently is preferable to phone calls that result in voice-mail messages, which may be perceived as less personal or even as a HIPAA violation (if overheard or retrieved by others). These are just a few of the pros associated with patient-related, provider e-mails; however, as you likely realize, there are a number of negative aspects to patient-related e-mail communication.

Cons of Patient-Related E-mails

1. Provider has no control over potential forwarding of e-mails.
2. Legal issues (see Chapter 7).
3. Unlike phone conversations, e-mails can be printed out and saved as a permanent record of communication (this can be both positive and negative).
4. Like regular mail, misaddressed messages can create embarrassment and potential HIPAA violations.
5. Risk of miscommunication and lack of immediate feedback to a patient's concerns or misunderstandings.
6. Patient messages can become too lengthy and/or too frequent.

While there are a number of reasons to utilize patient-related e-mail communication, there are some very important concerns you need to consider and assess. One of the most important e-mail issues is the lack of control any e-mail sender has over the eventual forwarding of her or his message. Most of us have inadvertently hit the "reply to all" button, or clicked on the wrong e-mail address and realized after the fact that a message has been sent to an unintended recipient. While this may simply require more careful attention on the part of the sender, the reality is that once a recipient has an e-mail, she or he can forward it to whomever, and the sender has no control and likely will be unaware of the action. Therefore, the admonishment, "don't put anything in an e-mail you wouldn't want the world to see," is a great policy for healthcare providers to adhere to. A good rule of thumb is do not put any specifics in an e-mail that your patient would not want others to know. Therefore, you might feel comfortable stating, "your lab tests were normal," in an e-mail, but not, "your pregnancy test was negative." Also, remember that while you should never make derogatory comments about a patient, you would certainly not want to do so in an e-mail to a colleague that could be discoverable if a legal action results some time in the future.

Every provider has to weigh the positive and negative communication that can result from the use of patient-related e-mail. Johnson (2007) summarizes the situation stating, "when advice is offered via e-mail, a duty may be created and there will be a written record of how that duty was discharged" (p. 30). The important thing is for providers to understand the pros and cons associated with patient-related e-mail communication and to use that knowledge to make the best decision about its use for themselves and their patients. For more information, please refer to Chapter 7 and the American Medical Association's Communication Guidelines (2002) for e-mail use. It is great food for thought no matter what your profession.

Websites and Social Networks

As with e-mail use, providers need to understand that information posted on a website or in a social network has the potential for worldwide access. Therefore, if you would not normally communicate a message in writing, you probably should not be posting it in cyberspace. A personal or corporate website may be completely appropriate for your goals; however, you want to make sure that nothing posted on the Internet could be construed as medical advice. Information about you or your practice (location, hours, and so forth) should be of interest to your patients and family members, but disease and potential treatment discussions are likely best left for face-to-face discussions with patients.

Similarly, comments about patients or events at your workplace made on social networking pages, even if they do not include patient's names, may still be construed as HIPAA violations. For example, posting a nonspecific comment on your Facebook page about a drunken patient, even without a name, could result in a HIPAA violation if another patient who happened to be in the ED at the same time puts your statement together with the patient she or he saw. Or perhaps, you post a staged photo that is intended to be funny (for example, staff drunk at work or sleeping), but your employer or your licensure review board may not find it so humorous.

It is best not to post anything on your corporate or personal website that in any way could be considered a medical opinion or a comment about a patient or could be potentially embarrassing to your employer or your professional credibility. As discussed throughout this text, authors cannot guarantee how some information will be perceived by unintended audiences, and with the mass appeal of websites (corporate, personal, and social networking sites), it is nearly impossible for providers–authors to assess all potential audience perceptions of various information.

In closing, if you are interested in creating a website, be aware that disclaimers are not always enough to protect providers from a malpractice suit. In fact, attorney and MD Patricia Recupero and Samara Rainey (2007) state, "simply posting a disclaimer may not prevent a malpractice action if the physician provides advice upon which the patient relies to his [or her] detriment" (p. 174). Remember to carefully assess any information posted online and to avoid any medical discussion that could be construed as advice. The authors go on to discuss how posting links to other websites can be problematic, as well as receiving money for banner advertisements of pharmaceutical companies and encouraging or suggesting requests for advice (p. 173). In addition, attorney Lee Johnson (2007) believes, "[providers] with websites that attract patients nationwide must make sure that their malpractice insurance covers activities in other states" (p. 30). The bottom line is, if you are thinking about a website, do your research, get legal advice, understand the realities involved in such a venture, and manage your risk.

REFERENCES

American Medical Association. (2002). *Advocacy resources: Guidelines for physician–patient electronic communications*. Retrieved on July 10, 2009, from http://www.ama-assn.org/ama/pub/about-ama/our-people/member-groups-sections/young-physicians-section/advocacy-resources/guidelines-physician-patient-electronic-communications.shtml.

Callen, J., Alderton, M., & McIntosh, J. (2008). Evaluation of electronic discharge summaries: A comparison of documentation in electronic and handwritten discharge summaries. *International Journal of Medical Informatics, 77*, 613–620.

Childs, D., Chang, H., & Grayson, A. (2009, January 9). *President-Elect urges electronic medical records in five years: Companies scramble to develop, docs slow to adopt.* Retrieved on February 20, 2009, from http://abcnews.go.com/Health/President44/Story?id=6606536&page=1.

Franklin, B. (1754). *Some account of the Pennsylvania Hospital: From its first rise to the beginning.* Philadelphia: Franklin & Hall.

Johnson, L. (2007, August 3). Malpractice consult: Patient e-mail perils. *Medical Economics, 84*(9), 30.

Recupero, P., & Rainey, S. (2007, June). Websites and e-mail in medical practice: Suggestions for risk management. *Medicine & Health/Rhode Island, 90*(6), 173–177.

T System. (2008). T System for physicians: Features and samples. Retrieved on March 6, 2009, from http://www.tsystem.com/Paper-Charting-Solutions/emergency-physicians/features.asp.

Chapter 7

Legal Considerations for Authors of Patient Records

by Canera L. Pagano, RN, JD

Overview

The patient record provides a valuable source of information for various individuals and entities that need access to the contents of the record. Patient records are utilized by insurance companies to substantiate billing for treatment and procedures as well as to establish a basis for medical therapy and future treatment. Patient records are also relevant in legal actions including personal injury suits, criminal cases, workers' compensation actions, disability determinations, and medical malpractice claims.

Physicians and other healthcare providers rely on the accuracy of the information contained in patient records when making preventative and treatment decisions. The patient record serves as a permanent record of the information obtained and the therapies provided and the role of each caregiver in the patient's course of treatment. As such, the patient record is often a critical piece of evidence when a patient claims she or he was harmed by the negligence of a physician, nurse, or other provider.

The contents of the patient record can seriously impact the defensibility of a claim of medical malpractice. If a record is poorly maintained, has gaps in documentation or missing pages, is illegible, contains unsanctioned abbreviations or obliterations and/or erasures, the quality of care provided is frequently called into question. Combine a poorly maintained patient record with a poor patient outcome, and you have a recipe for a medical malpractice action that will disrupt your life and may have serious consequences for your career.

How are medical malpractice risks, the Joint Commission, and Medicare regulations interrelated?

_____

_____

_____

Medical Malpractice

Malpractice has been defined as "unskillful practice resulting in injury to the patient, a failure to exercise the required degree of care, skill and diligence under the circumstances" (Furrow, Greaney, Johnson, Stoltzfus, & Schwartz, 2000, p. 264). Healthcare providers, lawyers, and accountants are all members of professions who can be held liable for malpractice. The burden of proof in a medical malpractice action lies with the injured patient. Unlike criminal cases, which require proof beyond a reasonable doubt, the level of proof in a malpractice case is considerably less and only requires proof of negligence by a preponderance of the evidence. This merely means that the facts are more likely to support the versions of events in favor of the plaintiff, or patient, rather than the provider, or defendant. Given the low level of proof required in a malpractice action, the content of the patient record can easily tip the scales of justice one way or the other.

The importance of medical records is further heightened by the reality that it often takes years before a medical malpractice action is filed and winds its way through the litigation process to trial. Memories fade over time, and as a result, healthcare providers have to rely on the documentation of events that occurred years prior regarding care and treatment given at the time. Therefore, the record should tell the story of the information obtained and the care provided to the patient. It is also important that the documentation be in chronological order, accurate, and thorough, thus demonstrating that the standard of care was met by the provider–author.

The Joint Commission requires the maintenance of adequate patient records. This organization also mandates that documentation in patient records be accurate, adequate, and timely with information readily available and accessible for prompt retrieval and stored in a confidential and secure manner (Furrow et al., 2000, p. 144). Similarly, the federal government's Medicare program, as a condition of participation, requires hospitals to have a medical record service and a patient record to be maintained for every individual evaluated or treated in the hospital. Medicare also requires the patient record to be accurately written, promptly completed, properly filed, retained, and accessible. In addition, documentation in the patient record should justify admission and continued hospitalization, support the diagnosis, and describe the patient's progress and response to medical treatment. All entries must be legible, complete, and authenticated and dated promptly by the person, identified by name and discipline, responsible for ordering, providing, or evaluating the service furnished (42 C.F.R. §482.24).

Most hospitals, long-term care, or other facilities are required to have policies and procedures regarding the maintenance of patient records and documentation. It is important to know and be familiar with your organization's policy. Among other things, the policies typically address how to handle late entries or errors in the record. In addition, there may be a list of abbreviations that have been approved by the organization for use in the patient record. Failure to follow, or to be familiar with, an institution's documentation policy can raise questions regarding the accuracy and completeness of the record and/or the competence of the provider.

Both the Joint Commission and Medicare emphasize that documentation contained in patient records should have the following basic characteristics in that they should be timely, accurate, complete, and legible. As a starting point, ensuring that your documentation meets these basic requirements can go a long way in helping you prevent or defend against a medical malpractice claim.

How does the timing of documentation impact the author's credibility?

_____

_____

_____

Timeliness

All care or treatment provided and interactions with physicians or other healthcare providers should be documented in the record as soon as possible. The entry should contain the date and time the entry was authored in the patient record. It is not always possible to document care and treatment contemporaneously, and as a result, it is vital to document events as soon as possible. If you wait until the end of a shift to complete documentation, it often leads to incomplete and inaccurate patient records. An example of a timely entry might appear as follows (handwritten in the original):

9/12/06, 6:30 p.m.

At 5:45 p.m., Mr. Smith ambulated to the nurse's station and back to his room without difficulty. He denied shortness of breath or chest pain.

Michael _____, RN

Such a simple entry provides a wealth of information that may be beneficial in the future if there is ever a question regarding the level of activity or condition of this patient. We know, from looking at the entry, when and at what time the nurse completed the documentation. We also know what time the patient was up and ambulating in the hallway, how far he ambulated, and how he tolerated the event. We are told the identity of the person who authored the entry as well as the author's profession. All of these facts may be relevant in the future and assist in the defense of a claim of malpractice.

All entries in the patient record should contain the complete date, which consists of the month, day, and year, as well as the time the note or entry was made including designating a.m. or p.m. if military time is not being used. While that sounds fairly basic, the failure to include any one of those elements can be problematic when trying to recreate a timeline of care in the event of a lawsuit. Failure to document the complete date is especially problematic in a long-term care setting where patients may be residents of a facility for several years. As a result, there may be more than one progress note, nurse's note, or flow sheet for a particular date in question. If the date is incomplete, for instance, if there is no year recorded, it may be difficult, if not impossible, to determine where in the timeline certain events occurred or care was rendered.

In addition to recording the complete date, all entries should have the author's full signature, which includes the first and last name of the provider as well as his or her professional abbreviation (RN, CNA, MD, PA, etc.). If only initials are used, then there should be a place in the patient record where the full name and corresponding initials are documented in order to identify providers at a later time. The designation of the author's profession, via an abbreviation, after the signature allows readers to know which disciplines were involved in the patient's treatment, such as doctors, nurses, physical therapists, pharmacists, and/or nutritionists.

You forgot to document something related to your patient. How would you do it the following day, or would you just leave it out and why?

_____

_____

_____

Late Entries

A late entry in a patient record is documentation of a treatment, response to treatment, or other event that is out of sequence and not in chronological order. It is important to document a late entry in accordance with your organization or facility's standard or policy. Typically, late entries are designated as such in the record by noting that the documentation is a "Late Entry" with the date and time when the addendum was made. Some policies direct that the date on which the late entry was made be circled in order to draw attention to the fact that the note is out of sequence.

Using the previous example, if the nurse forgot to document that Mr. Smith ambulated in the hallway on September 12, 2006, she may document the information as follows:

9/13/06, 3:00 p.m.

Late Entry for 9/12/06 at 5:45 p.m., Mr. Smith ambulated to the nurse's station and back to his room without difficulty. He denied shortness of breath or chest pain. Michael _____, RN

When documenting a late entry in a patient record, it is important to follow the policy of your facility or organization. Remember that as a general rule, late entries in a patient's record can raise questions regarding the reliability of the information documented and the credibility of the provider–author. For this reason, all too often late entries in patient records are looked upon as self-serving. Can you tell if the following is a true late entry or a self-serving statement of care after an untoward event?

1/8/03, 12:28 p.m.

Patient found by CNA on floor lying on his back complaining of pain in his left hip. Left leg shortened and externally rotated with positive pedal pulse. Patient stated that he fell when trying to get out of bed to go to the bathroom. Michael _____, RN

1/9/03, 08:00 a.m.

Late Entry for 1/8/03, 10:30 a.m., instructed patient to call for assistance when getting out of bed. Both side rails are up and call bell is within reach. Reviewed with patient how to use call bell and return demonstration was appropriate. Jane _____, RN

QUESTIONS

1. How would you evaluate this late entry?

   _____

   _____

   _____

2. Since the patient fell on 1/8/03, how did that event change your evaluation of the late entry? Why?

   _____

   _____

   _____

3. How does the reader's use of the record likely affect his or her assessment of the late entry, for example, a healthcare provider versus a malpractice attorney reader?

   _____

   _____

   _____

The above documentation may very well be true and accurate; however, the late entry raises questions with regard to the safety teaching provided and when or if it was communicated to the patient prior to the fall. If the patient should file a lawsuit as a result of his fall, his attorney will try to convince a jury that the late entry was only written after the fact out of fear of a lawsuit and as an attempt to lay blame on the patient for his own injuries. That is not to say that late entries should never be made; if the teaching or treatment was actually provided, then it should be documented in accordance with the facility or organization's policy. However, the situation in the example above is all too common and stresses the importance of timely and complete documentation.

What are some specific things you can include in your documentation to make your record more accurate and complete?

_____

_____

_____

Accurate and Complete Records

Documentation of medical treatment is a continuum. Providers increase their knowledge of the patients' information, conditions, treatments, and progress based on their own assessment as well as on the documentation of prior interactions, therapies, and outcomes. Proper decision making can only be expected to occur when patient records are accurate and complete. Documentation is the prime method by which various disciplines in health care communicate with one another and with other readers (for example, insurance companies and malpractice attorneys), highlighting the importance of accurate and complete patient records.

The significance of accurate and complete documentation is reflected in its ability to communicate a breadth of information obtained from and with the patient, as well as from other providers and the author's observations, assessments, and decisions. Whenever possible the patient's own words in quotation marks should be used. Quoting the patient directly in the record provides clear documentation of the patient's complaints, statements, and so forth, and provides a more objective foundation for evaluating the provider's assessment and plan of treatment. In addition, using patient quotes can provide the reader with other vital information, such as the patient's attitude, level of cooperation, and credibility (Teichman, 2000).

Quoting the patient can also help assist other individuals who may be facing litigation resulting from injuries to the patient not related to medical care and treatment. For example, if a patient complains of injury to his or her ankle, a statement by the patient that "I twisted my ankle 2 days ago after tripping over an area rug" will be more beneficial in defeating a claim that the patient slipped and fell in an icy parking lot 2 days ago than a statement of "pt. complains of right ankle pain for 2 days." Documenting how and when the patient was injured can help healthcare providers–authors avoid having to testify years later about the contents of their documentation concerning the patient's injury.

When documenting your observations or assessments, pejorative or judgmental statements should not be used. Although it seems to be common sense, do not include terms, such as obnoxious, rude, crazy, or drunk, in your subjective assessment of the patient. Using pejorative statements makes you appear unprofessional and judgmental. In addition, such descriptors do not allow other providers to gauge if there is an improvement or deterioration in the patient's condition. Instead, document your objective observations of the patient's behavior or condition, for example, "the 19-year-old male smelled of alcohol and had slurred speech." These objective findings can be reassessed by other providers, and any changes further documented.

In addition to steering clear of negative comments about patients, negative statements about other providers should be avoided as well. Documentation of conflicts with staff members, perceived incompetence of other providers, and staffing problems do not belong in the patient record. Recording such incidents and opinions only reinforces the impression that the provider is not a professional or may offer further ammunition as to why the overall care provided was substandard. Similarly, blaming another provider for his or her actions or decisions in the patient record should be avoided. Documentation that blames another provider or discipline for patient injury raises questions about the care rendered not only by the accused provider but by the author as well. Often, blame is asserted in a patient record in an effort to deflect inquiry into the care provided by the author; this is especially true when two different disciplines provide overlapping care. For example, "the nurses applied the bandage too tightly" may or may not be true, but it does not belong in the patient record. If the author did not witness who applied the dressing, she or he cannot be certain who actually performed the action. Instead, documenting the objective findings, "the patient's leg was swollen and erythematous distal to the bandage around her left mid-calf."

Accurate and complete patient records should not have any gaps in documentation. The record should be chronological and sequential. A gap in the record raises questions regarding the integrity of the document and concerns that information has been deleted, left out, or intentionally destroyed. When litigation is threatened or a lawsuit is filed, it is important to secure the patient record in order to preserve the evidence contained in the chart. Lost records can not only create a negative perception of the provider but liability as well.

In *Keene v. Brigham & Women's Hospital, Inc.*, 785 N.E.2d 824 (2003), the Massachusetts Supreme Court affirmed the decision of the lower court in granting summary judgment as a sanction for losing the patient record. It was claimed that the hospital failed to timely treat and diagnose meningitis in an infant resulting in severe disability. Eighteen hours of notes and documentation were missing from the record, and, as a result, the family was only able to identify the hospital as a defendant in the action. This was a critical time period in the treatment of this patient, and the Massachusetts Supreme Court found that it was not clear if the loss or destruction of the record was intentional or not. However, the loss of the information was catastrophic to the claims of the child and parents as they were deprived of the identities of the healthcare providers involved.

Documentation that fails to provide a clear picture of the patient's condition can also create liability. In *Lama v. Borras* 16 F.3d 473 (1994), a hospital's policy of charting by exception resulted in substandard record keeping and a delay in diagnosis and treatment of a patient's infection. In the Lama case, the nursing staff charted by exception, whereby notes were made only when there was an important change in the patient's condition. The court determined that this intermittent charting failed to provide the sort of continuous danger signals that would spur early intervention and treatment by a physician. A former nurse testified that when charting by exception, she would not record a patient's complaint of pain if she did not administer medication or only administered an over-the-counter pain reliever. As a result, the nursing staff did not record important signs and symptoms that would have likely prompted a diagnosis of infection (Tammelleo, 1994). This case presents a situation in which the patient record failed to tell a story and resulted in injury to the patient. It is also illustrative of the importance of the accuracy and completeness in documentation as a tool for effective communication.

How do you think your handwriting might impact your malpractice risk?

_____

_____

_____

Legible Records

Perhaps you have joked with a colleague or friend and commented "with handwriting like that you could be a doctor." Illegible patient records are no laughing matter, and poor penmanship is not limited to physicians. Illegible records cause problems for other providers who are trying to care for patients, as well as for attorneys who are trying to defend claims of malpractice. However, it is important to realize that illegible records include not only poor penmanship but also the use of unsanctioned abbreviations, obliterations, erasures, and writing in the margins.

If handwriting is not neat and clear, mistakes can be made such as medication errors and/or procedures performed on incorrect body parts. In addition, as time passes and memories fade, it may become impossible for the author to decipher his or her own handwriting. One court found that when the record was illegible or comprehensible only to the creator, the probative value of the record was minimal to nonexistent (*Wilson v. Bodian*, 130 A.D.2d 221, 1987). When records are illegible, there is a concern that they may not be admitted into evidence and, therefore, may not be available for use in support of the provider's defense.

The Wilson case is also illustrative of another problem with regard to legible records, and that includes the use of abbreviations in documentation.

In *Wilson*, the court found that at the time it was used, there was no proof that the abbreviation "BX" for biopsy was well known and usual in the medical community. Such a finding by a court could prohibit a provider from using the record to demonstrate that a particular test or treatment was ordered or provided. It is important to limit abbreviations to only those that are sanctioned by the facility or organization where you work. In addition, the Joint Commission has a list of abbreviations that are not to be used (the Joint Commission Official "Do Not Use" List). Abbreviations in documentation have fallen out of favor as they are subject to multiple interpretations depending on the reader (for example, Pt for patient and for physical therapy, or BS for breath sounds and bowel sounds). In addition, abbreviations can lead to errors in transcription (verbal orders and dictated reports), which can harm the patient if the wrong dose or schedule of treatment is interpreted.

Other problems that create illegible patient records are obliterations and erasures, which may appear to be an attempt to alter the document and cover up a mistake. If you have inadvertently documented something in the record that does not belong, a single line should be drawn through the improper documentation so that it can still be read, and the change should be dated and initialed. By properly correcting an error in documentation, you can avoid raising the suspicion that you are attempting to avoid liability by covering up a mistake.

Similarly, writing in the margins gives the impression that the record has been altered and documentation has been added after the fact. Furthermore, documentation in the margins may not photocopy. If additional information needs to be added, the facility's policy for late entries or addendums to the record should be followed.

Let us look at an example and try to apply this discussion of legal considerations to our analysis of a verbatim patient record.

Progress Note

Subj.: "I hurt all over doc."

Obj.: VS stable, lab WNL, lungs clear.

Imp: Cefoxitin appears to be working.

Rx: Continue Cefoxitin.

P.: Await C&S, recheck CBC tomorrow.

JB.

QUESTIONS

1. How would you evaluate this progress note?

   _____

   _____

   _____

2. How would you assess the timeliness of this entry?

   _____

   _____

   _____

3. What are your views on the accuracy and completeness of this documentation?

   _____

   _____

   _____

4. Are there legibility issues in this record? If so, what are they. If not, why?

   _____

   _____

   _____

5. Is this a timely or a late entry? Why?

   _____

   _____

   _____

6. Does this record accomplish the author's purpose and use for a progress note? If so, why? If not, why?

   _____

   _____

   _____

As you likely noted, this very brief progress note provides very few of the important elements discussed in this chapter. There is no date, and consequently, the author appears to expect readers to interpret the mere position of the entry in the record as a way to determine its date. However, that is risky for the author, and depending on the accuracy and timeliness of the entries prior to and following this entry, they may create more confusion than clarity. Each entry in a patient's record needs to be clearly dated (month, day, year). Because of the lack of a date, readers cannot determine from this document if this was a timely or late entry. Similarly, the accuracy of this record is called into question by its brevity and lack of clear information. For example, a quote from the patient is provided; however, the subjective information, the quote, and the impression "Cefoxitin appears to be working" seem to be contradictory. The patient's complaint is never explained to the reader, so these apparent conflicting accounts (patient's versus provider's impression) are left to the reader to resolve. It seems likely that the provider is basing his or her impression on the vital signs and lab data (which are not provided) but which apparently did not include a CBC, since the author intends to recheck that tomorrow.

From a legibility perspective, this record also creates malpractice risks by not clearly documenting who is authoring this progress note. Readers cannot tell if JB refers to an MD, DO, PA, or APRN. Or JB could be the initials of an intern, resident, or healthcare student. And as discussed, using abbreviations for the author's name is not a wise practice because other members of the team may have similar initials and it may create further confusion about the author of this document. In addition, while "WNL" may be an acceptable abbreviation for within normal limits, the lack of description about which lab tests were performed makes this abbreviation contribute to the confusion created by this entry.

It would seem very unlikely that the author of this progress note intended to create so many problems for readers. We can assume that the author's purpose for this record was to inform readers of the patient's status, based on the patient's current complaints, vital signs, laboratory tests, physical examination findings, and so forth; however, this document appears woefully short of attaining the author's goals and instead calls into question the provider's credibility. In order for a reader to use this document, the reader has to try to determine when it was authored and by whom, what lab tests were done, and how to reconcile the apparent conflict between the patient's quote and the provider's impression. And finally, the reader, in order to use this document effectively, has to guess at who actually authored it.

E-mail Communication

As technology advances, the manner in which we communicate with each other on a daily basis has the potential to work its way into the patient–provider relationship. This is especially true with e-mail communication. E-mail can be an efficient and cost-effective manner in which to interact with a patient; however, it is not without its perils from a medicolegal standpoint.

Patients and providers alike increasingly use e-mail as a means of communication. E-mail, however, tends to be less formal, and as a result, providers should use care when corresponding with patients over the Internet. Issues and areas of concern that are raised by patient-related e-mails include confidentiality, content, and record maintenance.

Because e-mail communication can and does concern all aspects of the patient's health care, confidentiality is critical. The Health Insurance Portability and Accessibility Act (HIPAA) applies to the content of e-mail communication that contains protected health information. Before a provider–author begins to interact with a patient via the Internet, a discussion should take place with the patient about the use of e-mail as a means of communication. Corresponding by e-mail may not be appropriate in certain situations such as when a patient shares a computer with another family member. In addition, e-mails may be inadvertently sent to the wrong recipient, or if sent to the patient through his or her employer's computer system, the e-mail may be available to the employer. It should be made clear to the patient that there is no way to guarantee confidentiality when communicating protected health information over the Internet and that there is a constant threat that the integrity of the system may be breached and the patient's information accessed. As a result, any conversation with a patient about the use of e-mail should also include a discussion of the safeguards instituted by the provider to ensure the confidentiality of the records, such as firewalls, encryption, and password protection of information (Recupero & Rainey, 2007). Like any conversation with a patient, the discussion regarding the use and appropriateness of e-mail as a means of communication between the provider and patient should be documented in the patient's record.

In addition to confidentiality, consideration should be given to the content of e-mail communication with patients. There are some aspects of medical care that are better left to face-to-face communication with the patient. Conveying the results of important lab tests or diagnostic studies are better-suited to in-person communication rather than e-mail format. Many aspects of medical treatment require in-depth discussions regarding treatment options and prognosis, which are not suitable to e-mail communication. Furthermore, communication by e-mail limits the ability of the provider to gauge the reaction of the patient and also limits the ability of the patient to gauge the level of compassion of the provider (Recupero & Rainey, 2007).

Similar to maintaining standard medical records, e-mail communication with patients also needs to be preserved. The e-mails should be printed out in paper format and kept in the chart or saved directly onto the server if electronic records are used. It is especially important to make sure that any reply to a patient e-mail is saved. Furthermore, if the provider requests a "read receipt" for e-mails with patients, that e-mail receipt should also be saved in the record as further evidence of when communication with a patient occurred.

As more and more patients and physicians use e-mail and the Internet as means of communication, lawyers increasingly ask for, or oftentimes subpoena, electronic records and electronic communication of healthcare providers. As with a paper record, once litigation is threatened or started, electronic records should be preserved and maintained. This means that hard drives should not be manipulated, erased, or removed from the computer. The Federal Rules of Civil Procedure have been amended to address electronic discovery. The rules set forth the requirement that small and large businesses and corporations preserve, maintain, collect, and produce electronically stored information that is potentially relevant to litigation. Under both federal and state law, a party to a lawsuit or threatened lawsuit has an affirmative duty to preserve potentially relevant information regarding the litigation. The duty to preserve applies to both paper and electronic records. The federal rule also provides for sanctions for failure to maintain electronic records (Federal Rules of Civil Procedure 34, 2009).

Electronic communication with patients is not without risk and is not a decision that should be taken lightly or made without a thorough discussion with the patient. There are many other issues related to patient-related e-mail and Internet communication that cannot be discussed here, and providers are encouraged to contact their risk managers or personal counsel for a more complete discussion of the risks and benefits of electronic interactions with patients.

Summary

Healthcare providers–authors have an onerous task—to communicate clearly, accurately, and completely in their patient records. And, this is expected despite current healthcare practices that provide far too little time for interviewing, examining, and assessing patient's complaints, problems, and wellness or illness. However, the obligation to document information in patient records is nonetheless a critical one for all healthcare providers. Without effective patient record keeping, providers–authors may find themselves not just trying to recall what they intended to communicate but defending what they did record or failed to document. In order to minimize your malpractice risk, use your documentation to help you care for your patients, to assist other providers in their treatment, and to ensure that, if necessary, the records illustrate and demonstrate the information obtained, your assessment, treatment decisions, and outcomes. To accomplish these important goals, know the policies and procedures for documentation at your institution(s) and use the following checklist for all your patient records to ensure that they meet the organization's and national standards:

- Timeliness
- Accuracy and completeness
- Legibility
- Late entries

Finally, before and when communicating with patients via e-mail, be sure to consider two key factors: "e-mail creates a written, signed, and dated document that can become evidence in a malpractice suit. . . . [and] advice based only on a patient's written description of symptoms might not be within the standard of care" (Johnson, 2007, p. 30). The ease of use associated with e-mail interactions should be thoughtfully weighed against the potential malpractice risks related to its use in patient-related communication.

REFERENCES

Federal Rules of Civil Procedure (2009). New York: Thomson West.

Furrow, B., Greaney, T., Johnson, S., Stoltzfus Jost, T., & Schwartz, R. (2000). *Health Law* (2nd ed.). Saint Paul, MN: West Group.

The Joint Commission (2005). Official do not use list. Retrieved on May 2, 2009, from http://www.jointcommission.org/NR/rdonlyres/2329F8F5-6EC5-4E21-B932-54B2B7D53F00/0/dnu_list.pdf.

Johnson, L. (2007, August 3). Malpractice consult: Patient e-mail perils. *Medical Economics, 84*(9), 30.

Keene v. Brigham & Women's Hospital, Inc., 785 N.E.2d 824 (2003).

Lama v. Borras, 16 F.3d 473 (1994).

Recupero, P., & Rainey, S. (2007, June). Websites and e-mail in medical practice: Suggestions for risk management. *Medicine & Health/Rhode Island, 90*(6), 173–177.

Tammelleo, D. (1994). Court holds "charting by exception" policy negligent: Case in point: *Lama v. Borras* 16 F. 2d 473 PR (1994). *Legal Lesson of the Month in Regan Report on Nursing Law, 34*, 12.

Teichman, P. (2000). Documentation tips for reducing malpractice risk. *Family Practice Management, 7*(3), 29–33.

Title 42: Public Health (2007). 42 C.F.R. §482.24. Condition of participation: Medical record services. Retrieved on 5/1/2009, from http://law.justia.com/us/cfr/title42/42-3.0.1.5.21.3.199.4.html.

Wilson v. Bodian, 130 A.D.2d 221 (1987).

Chapter 8

Practicing the Process

Skills Require Practice

Up to this point, we have discussed the authoring process, the content expected by readers, the importance of the context or the reason for creating the document, and the legal considerations for healthcare providers–authors. In addition, we have explored the importance of audience, purpose, and use analysis. However, as everyone who has authored any type of document realizes, there is a major difference between knowing what needs to be communicated and how to format a record and effectively meeting the reader's needs and the author's goals. In written or electronic communication, one of the best ways to improve your authoring skills is to practice them. That is the purpose of this chapter. The more you can build the habits necessary to improve your pre-authoring and re-authoring skills and decrease the time required to accomplish them, the more you will enhance the communication effectiveness of your patient records.

Because we are interested in practicing the authoring process, let us begin by examining the same data regardless of your profession. You will get an opportunity for profession-specific practice later on in this chapter. To start, please review the following data and try to examine it as if you had just obtained it from a patient.

A Patient's History

"My name is Helen Galag. I'm a 54-year-old married, white, female biology professor at Shanahan University. My husband works for the state department in Vietnam. I have 2 children, twins, who are sophomores at Shanahan. I've been running a fever, around 102, for the past 3 days, but the boys aren't sick. I don't hurt anywhere in particular, but ache all over. I'm not coughing, vomiting, urinating more frequently or burning when I urinate, and I don't have diarrhea. I do have high cholesterol, take a statin, a baby aspirin, and fish oil every day. I don't have any allergies, don't smoke, but I do have an occasional glass of wine. I've had my gallbladder and tonsils out and no other surgeries. My dad is still alive at 84, but my mom died at 80 from lymphoma, and I don't have any siblings."

Pre-Authoring Skills Application

Primary audience (based on your profession and patient's problem):

_____

_____

_____

Secondary audiences:

_____

_____

_____

_____

What additional history information would you like to have from this patient?

_____

_____

_____

_____

Based on the information presented, author a history for this patient.

_____

_____

_____

_____

_____

_____

_____

As you thought about this history and your documentation of it, what were the most critical elements of the patient's narrative for you to communicate to your primary and secondary readers and why?

_____

_____

_____

_____

_____

_____

_____

_____

As you may recall, interviewing a patient and/or family member are generally best accomplished through the use of open-ended questions that allow the interviewee to tell his or her story (usually a narrative, like that of Ms. Galag). Then, you can use closed-ended questions (how high was your fever, for how many days, did you have blood in your urine, and so forth) to gain more detailed information and to clarify any unclear or missing data (Pagano, 2010, p. 69). However, based on the interviewee's narrative, how much of the following information, beyond her specific complaints and negative symptoms, did you find important to record?

- Patient's occupation
- Her husband's occupation
- Patient's past, family, and social histories

As you considered the breadth of information that you were presented, you had to make some very important decisions as an author:

1. What information was critical to the further evaluation of this patient?
2. What data were readers going to expect to aid in their assessment of her complaint and your evaluation of it?
3. Should you merely record everything she told you?

While these questions are critical to your pre-authoring analyses, it is unlikely that you would want to record everything as told to you; for one reason, it is not all needed, and for another, your role here is to record the information that is important to your decision making (and consequently, to your readers' analyses of your patient's condition and your decision making). Therefore, let us list the critical information to record:

- Name
- Age

- Chief complaint
- Details about complaint (chronology, level of fever, positive and negative symptoms)
- Key elements of the past medical, family, and social histories
- Patient's occupation
- Husband's job

Did you include the patient's and her husband's jobs in your history? Why or why not?

_____

_____

_____

As you assessed this history, you likely recognized very quickly the difficulty it presents for a healthcare provider. First, a fever of unknown origin (FUO) is a very complicated and complex problem to evaluate. However, Ms. Galag did provide some helpful information. You can assume (eventually you should ask to confirm) that she took her temperature and how elevated it was (since she told you a specific number) and for how many days. She also told you in a general way that she does not have a sore throat, chest pain, abdominal pain, and so forth (clearly, you would want to explore each of these areas in much greater detail with specific closed-ended questions). She further discussed the fact that she had no nausea and no urinary tract symptoms. Therefore, you can at least tentatively reduce the likelihood the fever is caused by a typical upper respiratory infection (URI), gastrointestinal condition (GI; gastritis or gastroenteritis), or urinary tract infection (UTI). So, your readers would definitely want to know this information. But as you begin to reorder in your mind the potential etiologies for her fever, you likely would want to at least consider the fact that her mother had a lymphoma. You would want to know more about her occupation as a biologist—any animal bites or exposure to animals, pathogens, and microbes. Perhaps, even more of a factor is Mr. Galag's career as a state department official in Vietnam.

What might your readers want to know about the patient and her husband's job posting in Vietnam?

_____

_____

_____

With a working diagnosis of FUO, based on this brief history, would you, as the healthcare provider, and subsequently the readers of your patient record, not want to know when Ms. Galag was last in Vietnam visiting her husband? As you may know, one of the major cautions for travelers to Southeast Asia is the risk of malaria, which could cause her fever. In addition, of course you would want to explore any recent history of tick or mosquito bites in this country, along with the aforementioned in-depth discussion about her job as a biologist and its potential relevance to her FUO.

The point of this is not to discuss the entire review of systems that you would want to explore with this patient but instead to highlight how a patient's or even a spouse's occupation may seldom be necessary to document in a patient's record. However, based on the patient's complaints, symptoms, and circumstances, you as the provider would be expected to explore all of these areas to rule in or rule out potential etiologies, and your readers will want to do the same and to at least be assured that you thoroughly explored them.

Remember, what you do not include in a patient record does not mean you did not do it, or ask it, but it does mean that readers have no way of knowing that you did it or asked it. So, a lack of communication is frequently perceived by readers as an author's lack of information. If you do not tell the reader that Ms. Galag had not been to Vietnam in 2 years and had no history of malaria, the reader will not know these facts, or more importantly perhaps, not know that you asked about them. The same is true regarding her risk of exposure at work.

Let us have a word about interviewing patients and/or family members. Try to continually remind yourself that you need as much data as possible to make the most informed diagnostic and treatment decisions you can. And while it is true that you will obtain a plethora of information from objective findings—vital signs, lab tests, x-rays—providers, since the time of Imhotep in ancient Egypt and Hippocrates in Greece (du Pré, 2005, pp. 25–28), have recognized the distinct advantage of communicating with patients about their complaints, history, and situation. It is the major distinguishing characteristic between veterinary and human health care.

Communicating What You See and Hear

Providers generally get to dialogue with patients and, in most cases, gather key data to include in their analyses. But as a provider–author, you need to recognize that the benefit of human communication with a patient to your decision making is also necessary for your primary and secondary readers. Therefore, just as you mentally assessed Ms. Galag's narrative for details that would be important to your information gathering, your readers are likely using that same process to try to understand and replicate your analyses and decisions.

Skills Application

1. Go to a window and look around outside; give yourself a minute or two to observe all that you can see. Now, in the space below (and without looking back out the window), in as much detail as possible describe in a narrative (not list) exactly what you saw and its relationship to the things around it.

_____

_____

_____

_____

_____

_____

_____

_____

_____

2. What did you find difficult about authoring this narrative about what you saw? Why?

_____

_____

_____

3. Turn on your TV or your radio to a channel with dialogue (no voiceless music); be sure it is loud enough so that you can clearly hear it. With the sounds in the background, look around your room and observe everything you can see. Now, in the space below, document what you saw in as much detail as possible. Remember to author your document so that the reader will be oriented to the spatial arrangement of everything you

describe. Try not to look back at the room while you are writing this (use memory only).

_____

_____

_____

_____

_____

_____

_____

_____

_____

4. Now, read over your outside narrative (Question No. 1), then go to the window and compare what you documented with what you see. Be sure to examine the clarity of the description, the spatial arrangement of the objects to each other, dimensions, and so forth. What do you see that is effectively communicated? What do you see that is not effectively communicated? How different do you think it would be if you were an objective reader (not the author) analyzing this narrative against the view outside?

_____

_____

_____

_____

5. Do the same analysis of the narrative you authored about your room. What do you see that is effectively communicated? What do you see that is not effectively communicated? How different do you think it would be if you were an objective reader (not the author) doing this assessment?

_____

_____

_____

_____

6. What did you notice about the accuracy of the details and the descriptions (spatial, etc.) in the two different narratives? Was one more effective at accurately communicating what you observed? If so, what were the distinctions, and why do you think there was a difference between the two?

_____

_____

_____

_____

_____

7. What difference(s), if any, did the TV or radio dialogue in the background make in your documentation of what you observed and why?

_____

_____

_____

_____

_____

What did you discover through these exercises? How much stuff you have in your room? Hopefully, you recognize the reason for these types of authoring process exercises. One of your roles as a healthcare provider is to interview patients and/or their families, to perform some type of examination or evaluation, and to document your findings. The purpose of the exercises you just completed was to illustrate the difficulties, not just in recalling what you observed to document, but communicating what you observed in a manner that ensures that your readers get to *see* what you saw—that you replicate what you observed, and you report it in such a way that readers are clear where the laceration, tumor, or lesion is on the patient's body (spatially, dimensionally, and so forth). For example, if you had difficulty differentiating in your narrative for Question No. 1 above between five trees, how will you be able to describe a patient's five nevi or three lacerations? The process for communicating what you observed to readers so they can see what you saw is the same for your room, the outside, a pediatric patient, or a trauma victim. You have to first increase your powers of observation by focusing on the details of what you are viewing and then on how to communicate those details so that the reader can see them as well.

However, as you know, in American culture, we tend not to stare at people, especially strangers or nonintimates, so we are, for the most part, unaccustomed, and perhaps even uncomfortable, focusing on the details of another person's face or body while we talk with him or her (Trenholm & Jensen, 2008, pp. 63–66). Therefore, while you are trying to overcome the discomfort of staring at someone, you are also trying to maintain eye contact as much as possible, because we recognize the value we place on eye contact in this culture. And you are trying to listen to what the other person is saying while you are analyzing all the information you are assimilating and trying to determine what questions to ask, what tests to order, and so forth. Perhaps you found that just having the TV or radio on while you were trying to observe and document what was in your room was distracting. That noise, as communication researchers describe it, interferes with your listening abilities, but it can also hinder your retention of information, recall, and communication (Pearson, Nelson, Titsworth, & Harter, 2003, p. 19). And yet, how many healthcare settings are void of background noise from other conversations, overhead announcements, machinery, and the like? However, that does not even cover the noise that is created in your brain when you are trying to analyze incoming data and to develop new questions, diagnoses, and treatment options. All of these etceteras are what make it difficult to not just recall what you observed and heard but what you are able to document in your patient record. Therefore, it is vitally important for you to recognize these inherent difficulties for providers–authors. You have to gather information, and at the same time, analyze that data, use your analyses to seek additional data, and then document what you saw, heard, and deduced in a format that is clear and concise and effectively communicates to readers.

Now that we have explored some of the difficulties with information gathering, let us return to practicing the authoring process. You should interview and examine a fellow student or an assigned patient. Try to encourage your interviewee to use a narrative to describe her or his problem or situation and then, once it has been fully described, use closed-ended questions to clarify, explore details, and quantify (Pagano, 2010). If you have not authored many patient records, you may want to take a break and note the key findings from your interview, using quotes from the interviewee wherever possible. Then, you can do your objective assessment or treatment (based on your profession and role). Finally, for the purpose of practicing the process, spend a few minutes transcribing your pre-authoring analyses for this document, then authoring, re-authoring, and proofreading it.

Skills Application

1. Who is included in your anticipated audience for this patient record (primary and secondary readers)?

   Primary readers:

   _____

   _____

Secondary readers:

_____

_____

_____

2. What are the purposes for authoring this record?

_____

_____

3. What is your desired use for this document?

_____

_____

4. Which and how much content are needed to fulfill the audience, purpose, and use needs for this patient record?

_____

_____

_____

_____

5. In the space below, or on an additional page(s) if needed, author your profession-specific patient record based on your interview, exam, and/ or treatment, and your pre-authoring analysis (format and organize as appropriate for your profession and the type of document being created).

_____

_____

_____

_____

_____

_____

_____

_____

_____

_____

_____

Next, you need to re-author and review the document you just completed. So first, reread your pre-authoring goals related to you audience, purpose, use, and content analyses. Then, compare what you authored to those goals and make changes wherever you need to (use a single horizontal line to draw through the word[s] you want to change so the word[s] beneath the line can still be seen, then make any changes above the line, for instance, [corrected words ~~incorrect words~~]) in order to ensure effective communication and goal attainment. If you do not want to delete–revise, but instead add words, you should use a caret (see example that follows) to indicate you are adding new material to the sentence (new words ∧new words) and place it where it should be incorporated, but above the current line.

Finally, you should proofread your document (preferably with a little time—the more, the better between when you authored it and proofread it) to ensure there are no typos ("there" instead of "their"), misspelled words ("alot" instead of "a lot"), missing words, or formatting issues that need to be corrected. When you are satisfied that your document matches your pre-authoring goals, communicates effectively, enhances your professional credibility, and meets the readers' needs–expectations, then you should date and sign it.

This is one example of how you should practice the authoring process. However, the more you can practice your pre-authoring and re-authoring skills, the faster and more efficient and effective you will become. Also, writers need feedback, so seek out readers to provide you with an objective assessment of what you have communicated. As we noted earlier in this text, authors create documents for readers, so you need to understand where your perceptions of effective communication differ from your readers to reassess and ensure a better outcome for your readers, your patients, and yourself as the provider–author.

REFERENCES

du Pré, A. (2005). *Communicating about health: Current issues and perspectives* (2nd ed.). New York, NY: McGraw-Hill.

Pagano, M. P. (2010). *Interactive case studies in health communication.* Sudbury, MA: Jones & Bartlett.

Pearson, J., Nelson, P., Titsworth, S., & Harter, L. (2003). *Human communication.* Boston, MA: McGraw-Hill.

Trenholm, S., & Jensen, A. (2008). *Interpersonal communication* (6th ed.). New York, NY: Oxford.

Chapter 9

Analyzing Patient Records

What Works and What Needs Work

Now that we have discussed the authoring process and practiced it, the next step in authoring is to examine some sample patient records and to try to analyze what works in terms of the audience, purpose, and use for the document and what needs work. It is well documented that good authors are good readers. That is because the more you understand about how a piece of writing communicates and what makes it more or less effective, the easier it is for you to assess your own documents and revise them. So, let us practice the art of reading and analyzing.

Nurse's Note

0800–   Awake, eating breakfast. Oriented x3, skin W/D, no S.O.B. noted, O2 off. Crackles noted RML and crackles noted on LLL. Abd. soft with active BS. HLN intact to LFA site clear. Pedal pulses + bilat. Resp-nonlabored. No complaints.

1000–   Family here to visit patient.

1100–   ↑ to BR, gait steady.

1200–   Ate well. Bath done.

1300–   Ate lunch well.

1400–   SR ↑ & call light in reach wanting to take a nap. Sarah _____, RN

(Pagano & Ragan, 1992, p. 116)

QUESTIONS

1. Who are the primary and secondary audiences for this particular patient record?

   Primary: _____

   _____

   _____

   Secondary: _____

   _____

   _____

2. What are the nurse–author's likely purposes for authoring this document?

   _____

   _____

   _____

   _____

3. How did the author expect this Nurse's Note to be used by her intended audience?

   _____

   _____

   _____

4. Does anything in this record confuse you, or is there anything you are unclear about?

   _____

   _____

   _____

   _____

5. Based on this document, how would you evaluate the nurse–author's 8 hours of caring for this patient? Why?

   _____

   _____

   _____

   _____

6. Were you surprised that there was no mention of the patient's vital signs or pulse oximeter reading? Why do you think these values should be here or not be here, and why might they be missing?

_____

_____

_____

_____

7. How do you evaluate the abbreviations and acronyms used in this chart? Do they help the reader? Or, do they confuse the reader and create more questions?

_____

_____

_____

_____

We can surmise that the primary audience for this record includes the following:

- Nurses working with this patient
- Physicians, PAs, and/or APRNs caring for this patient
- Dietitians, pharmacists, physical therapists, respiratory therapists, and other allied healthcare providers treating this patient
- Nursing supervisors

And secondary audiences might be comprised of the following:

- Quality assurance staff
- Student nurses or other healthcare provider students
- Insurance case managers
- Joint Commission surveyors
- Hospital finance or billing staff
- Risk managers
- Malpractice attorneys

This record provides some very useful information. However, the majority of the data are included in the initial entry, and the remaining 6 hours of documentation are brief and do little to help the reader assess the patient's condition and the care provided. Clearly, some of the major purposes for authoring a Nurse's Note are to document the information shared between the patient and the author, as well as other subjective and objective assessments, and to record what interventions were supplied by the nurse–author and/or other healthcare providers during the author's shift. We can also assume that the author intends for the primary and secondary audiences to use this document as a source of information about the patient's evolving biological, sociological, and psychological wellness and/or illness. Clearly, this record provides some information about each of those areas, but it also lacks information that readers would expect and, as such, calls into question the author's abilities and/or credibility.

For example, the record does a good job of providing a date and time for the documentation and meets the timeliness objective discussed in Chapter 7. However, in terms of accuracy and completeness, there are a number of issues in this Nurse's Note:

1. Readers are told that the patient is eating breakfast, but there is no discussion of how much the patient consumed or what type of diet the patient is on.

2. The record describes the patient's pulmonary findings—"no S.O.B. noted, 02 off . . ."—then describes the abdominal exam, IV site, and the like, then returns to "Resp-nonlabored." However, this back-and-forth about the patient's respiration causes the reader to question why the entire exam was not discussed together. It also makes the reader curious and even unclear if the patient's breath and bowel sounds were really assessed, because we are told the patient was eating. Furthermore, there are no vital signs or pulse oximeter results reported or discussed for a patient who clearly has respiratory problems ("Crackles noted").

3. This apparent 8 hours of shift documentation were only provided at even hours. This regularly timed recording makes readers question what really happened and when? For example, was the family there at 1000 hours, or were they there sometime between 0900 and 1000 or 1000 and 1100? And if there is so much inaccuracy in the reporting of this information, how much of the objective data were inaccurate?

4. This record further suffers from a lack of specificity and detailed information. Readers are told that the patient "Ate well" at 1200, but then "Ate lunch well" at 1300. Again, these simple statements are confusing and call into question the author's credibility and professional abilities. Are these two different meals; if so why? And if not, then why are they repeated—just to fill in time slots? And once more, there is no quantification for the type of meal consumed or the amount. In addition, at 1200 the record states "Bath done," but it is also the same time the patient "ate lunch well," so unless the patient ate in the bath, readers do not know what to believe about this entry. But more importantly, from an activities of daily living (ADL) perspective, readers do not know if the patient bathed herself or himself or was bathed by family or staff.

5. Finally, in an era when the biopsychosocial approach to health communication is being advanced by many healthcare disciplines, this note provides no information about the patient's perceptions of his or her condition. There are no quotes from the patient in the 8 hours of

documentation, and other than "No complaints" and "wanting to take a nap," there are no references to the patient's state of mind, alertness, or communication.

This simple record, which should provide information for about 8 hours of care for a patient, does very little to help readers (primary and secondary) assess the nurse–author's information gathering, assessments, and interventions. Instead, the document is vague, brief, and provides little information directly related to the patient's biopsychosocial status, and what is presented creates more confusion than answers and calls the nurse–author's professional skills and credibility into question.

As our analyses continue to illustrate, patient records should not be merely viewed as a duty or an organizational requirement, but instead, should be perceived as an important communication tool that impacts a patient's care and the author's reputation. To demonstrate this further, let us examine another document to evaluate how patient records communicate to readers (typed in all caps in original).

Physical Therapy Outpatient Note

3/13/07

S: PT REPORTS HER TAILBONE IS FEELING "FINE, IT'S PRETTY GOOD ACTUALLY." PT'S C/C IS L HIP/GROIN PAIN EXACERBATED BY WT BEARING AND PROLONGED STANDING/WALKING. SHE ALSO C/O RECENT ONSET OF SEVERE NECK PAIN STATICALLY AND W/MOBILITY.

PT WAS 10 MIN LATE FOR THERAPY TODAY.

O: GAIT: DECREASED GAIT SPEED, DECREASED WB ON L LE, L SIDE LIMP

PAIN: 6/10 NECK AND L LE

RANGE OF MOTION L HIP: LIMITED SECONDARY TO PAIN AND INCREASED LE FLUID PT REPORTS RECENT INCREASE IN L LE EDEMA

STRENGTH (MMT):

	LEFT	RIGHT
HIP FLEX:	4–/5	5/5
HIP EXT:	4/5	5/5
KNEE FLEX:	4/5	4+/5
ANKLE DF:	5/5	5/5

WALKING SPEED: 1/30/07: 256 CM/SEC

3/13/07: 240 CM/SEC SECONDARY NEW ONSET
OF L GROIN/HIP PAIN

TREATMENT: (C) US TO R LEVATOR/UT 1.0 MHZ @ 1.02 W/CM2

MANUAL: STM/MFR TO (B) LEVATOR, R UT, (B) SCALENES

PASSIVE NECK MOBILITY

PASSIVE LEVATOR STRETCH

THER. EX: GLOBAL NECK FLEX STRETCH 2 X 30 SEC EA SIDE

A: TO DATE, PT HAS MET 50% OF HER STG'S AND HAS NOT MET HER OTHER STG'S SECONDARY TO LE PAIN. PT ALSO HAS NEW C/O CERVICAL SPASMS AND PAIN AND L LE/GROIN PAIN WHICH LIMITS HER AMBULATION AND STANDING TOLERANCE AT WORK.

PT'S ACTIVE AND PASSIVE HIP ROM IS LIMITIED SECONDARY TO PAIN AND INC IN L LE LYMPHEDEMA. PT'S INCREASING L LE SIZE RESULTS IN INCREASED LE WEIGHT CAUSING MULTIPLE GAIT DEVIATIONS AND INCREASED STRESS AND STRAIN ON HER LUMBAR SPINE.

PT REPORTED HER TAILBONE PAIN IS ALMOST UNNOTICABLE AT THIS POINT, SHE WAS FEELING MUCH BETTER UNTIL THIS WEEKEND WHEN HER L LE AND NECK BEGAN TO LIMIT HER FUNCTION. PT TO RETURN TO OCCUPATIONAL HEALTH NEXT WEEK.

P: RECOMMENDED CONTINUED PT 2X/WK FOR 4 MORE WEEKS FOR ACUTE CERVICAL MUSCLE SPASMS AND CONTINUE ASSESSMENT AND TREATMENT OF L LE DYSFUNCTION AND SUBSEQUENT PELVIC/HIP ANOMALIES.

IF YOU AGREE WITH THE PLAN OF CARE, PLEASE SIGN AND RETURN BY FAX.

_____   _____

_____, PT, MSPT   DATE

_____   _____

PHYSICIAN'S SIGNATURE   DATE

PT performed: + MANUAL THERAPY (15 MIN) MINUTES   :15

: + ULTRASOUND (15 MIN)   :8

: + THERAPEUTIC EXER (15 MIN)   :5

: + RE-EVALUATION PT OUTPT   :10

TOTAL MINUTES OF PT CARE   :38

QUESTIONS

1. Who are the primary and secondary audiences for this particular patient record?

   Primary: _____

   _____

   _____

   Secondary: _____

   _____

   _____

2. What are the physical therapist–author's likely purposes for creating this record?

   _____

   _____

   _____

   _____

3. How did the author expect this document to be used by her or his intended audiences?

   _____

   _____

   _____

4. Does anything in this record cause you confusion, or is there anything you are unclear about?

   _____

   _____

   _____

   _____

5. Based on this document, how would you evaluate the author's time working with this patient? Why?

   _____

   _____

   _____

   _____

6. Did you find this record to communicate the information you needed effectively? If yes, why? If no, why not?

_____

_____

_____

_____

This example of a Physical Therapy Outpatient Note is vastly different from the earlier Nurse's Note. Perhaps, even more surprising than the clarity of the information presented is the amount of information communicated in this record in about 38 minutes of interaction versus the 8 hours of provider–patient contact in the prior Nurse's Note. While it is true that sheer quantity is not the ultimate purpose or goal for authors of patient records, it should be obvious that the latter record does a much better job of documenting what transpired during the patient and therapist's time together than the Nurse's Note.

The physical therapist–author can be expected to have a primary audience that includes the occupational medicine provider who prescribed the patient's therapy, the physical therapists' manager or supervisor, an orthopedic surgeon, the patient's workers' compensation case manager, and the organization's billing staff. Secondary readers might include physical therapy students, Joint Commission reviewers, and workers' compensation attorneys. As such, this patient record does a very good job of meeting these diverse audiences' needs and expectations. First and foremost, the provider who prescribed the therapy can use this document to clearly assess the patient's status on the day of therapy, the treatments given, and the outcome of those procedures. In addition, the author's manager, the patient's case manager, and the billing staff can all clearly identify what was communicated, treatments performed, and the results of the interaction and therapy, as well as the author's recommendations for future treatments.

While this document is an excellent example of how to communicate with the intended audiences and how to meet or surpass their needs and/or expectations, there are a few areas that could be helped with revision. First, the all capitalized text is a bit disconcerting, especially since most readers perceive all caps to be intended as a nonverbal scream or a symbol for the author's anger. In addition, while many of the abbreviations used are standard across disciplines in health care (ROM, FLEX, EXT), several abbreviations are not standard and are, therefore, confusing and unclear to readers who are not physical therapists (and since the document requires a signature from a prescriber, it is clear that at least one of the primary readers is expected to be a nonphysical therapist). However, nonphysical therapists do not typically use abbreviations like "MMT" and "ANKLE DF." Furthermore, walking speed would be clearer if there was a range stated for the normal walking speed. In addition, the document uses "PT" to refer to the patient in the majority of the text, but to physical therapy in the closing: "P: Recommended continued pt 2x/wk for 4 more weeks. . . ." While it is true that the abbreviation PT can be used for both patient and physical therapy, it should not be used for both in the same document, and using uppercase PT to refer to physical therapy does make sense, but the entire document is capitalized, so it is impossible to differentiate between "pt" for patient and "PT" for physical therapy.

Finally, the statement "pt was 10 min late for therapy today" seems out of place in the Subjective section (unless there was a discussion by the patient of the reason for the tardiness). The Subjective section is intended for the patient's statements about her complaints and symptoms, not the author's observations about tardiness. But perhaps even more concerning is the paternalistic impression that statement implies. By stating the patient's late arrival in the record, the therapist is implying that the patient is behaving inappropriately, but without any further information, the reader does not know if this is a solitary or a recurring act. And it seems likely that the therapist would have been late from time to time, but it is extremely doubtful that the author would document his or her own lateness as part of the patient's record. Therefore, this simple sentence calls into question the patient's motivation to get well but also leads to questions about the author's motivation for including it without further explanation.

However, in spite of these few communication problems, the overwhelming majority of this document is very clear and effective in communicating the information needed by a reader. The author uses quotes from the patient to describe her subjective self-assessment of her recovery. In addition, a breadth of objective data are included ensuring that the reader draws the same conclusions about the patient's evaluation as the author. And the Assessment does a very good job of explaining the author's reasoning, recommendations, and decision making. The record is very detailed and specific about the physical therapist–author's assessment but also accounts for every minute of the time the patient spent in treatment. This information is invaluable to both primary and secondary readers including the workers' compensation case manager and the organization's billing office. The value of carefully documenting what the author learned from interacting with the patient, as well as from various tests and the results from therapy, makes it much more likely that readers will find the author credible and his or her recommendations professionally astute and correctly deduced.

Based on those two very different documents, let us turn our analysis to another type of patient record (this was a hand-signed document in the original). Please note that the "D: 1/4/84" below stands for the date the document was dictated and "T: 1/5/84" refers to the date the document was transcribed.

Discharge Summary

D: 1/4/84

T: 1/5/84

Summary: See history and physical on chart.

Laboratory:

Her febrile agglutinins were negative. Glucose 116. Repeated was 68. Calcium 8.6, phosphorous 2.9. She had had a past history of diabetes but it certainly didn't show up on this admission. Her lead, arsenic, and mercury levels were all within complete normal range. Her serum cortisol was negative. Chest, skull, CAT of head all negative. Barium enema normal urogram. Cervical findings showed some spurring. Bone scan was negative except for increased uptake in the left ankle. She had fracture of this in the past. Upper GI was negative with exception of very edematous mucosa in the proximal one-third suggesting postbulbar ulcer.

Dr. _____ and Dr. _____ called in consultation. She was thoroughly evaluated. It was out feeling that she had ulcer disease. She had diabetes by history. She had headaches probably cervical osteoarthritis and it was our feeling that possibly she should be seen in psychiatric consultation. She was approached with this and declined. She recommended antacids.

She will be discharged and this will be carried out.

_____, MD

QUESTIONS

1. Who are the primary and secondary audiences for this particular patient record?

    Primary: _____

    _____

    _____

    Secondary: _____

    _____

    _____

    _____

2. What are the author's likely purposes for authoring this record?

3. How did the author expect this document to be used by her or his in-
    tended audience?

4. Does anything in this record confuse you, or is there anything you are un-
    clear about?

5. Based on this document, how would you evaluate the physician–author's
    interactions, assessments, and decision making regarding this patient?
    Why?

6. Please list any necessary information that you find missing or confusing
    and state why?

As you analyzed this record, what were your thoughts regarding the various audiences for the document? Perhaps it would be helpful to first discuss the purpose and use for a discharge summary. The Joint Commission requirements state the following:

A concise discharge summary providing information to other caregivers and facilitating continuity of care includes the following:

- Reason for hospitalization
- Significant findings
- Procedures performed
- Care, treatment, and services provided
- Patient's condition at discharge
- Discharge information provided to the patient and family, as appropriate, to include:
  - Medications
  - Diet
  - Physical activity
  - Follow-up care
- Discharge information must be documented or dictated and authenticated within 30 days postdischarge (The Joint Commission Requirements, 2009, p. 1).

This summary of The Joint Commission requirements from a medical staff newsletter clearly states what is expected in a hospital discharge summary like the one shown above. While these expectations are from a time frame 20 years after the Discharge Summary was originally authored, the purpose and requirements for these documents have changed very little during this period. By its very title, providers–authors understand that the purpose for this document is to summarize the patient's hospitalization; however, as you can quickly assess, the patient record shown here does not meet these requirements or expectations.

First, the physician–author does not appear to understand who comprises the primary and secondary audiences for this document. We can assume that the primary readers of a discharge summary would at a minimum include the following:

- Other current healthcare providers for the patient
- Future healthcare providers for the patient
- The hospital's billing department
- The patient's insurance company, Medicare, and/or Medicaid

While secondary readers might include the following:

- Healthcare provider students
- The Joint Commission and/or Medicare surveyors
- Malpractice attorneys

All of these potential readers would be expected to know The Joint Commission requirements above, and therefore, the physician–author of this Discharge Summary should understand the importance of meeting these standards in terms of the purpose for his or her record. The problems we can identify in analyzing this patient record are that it does not meet these standards in any way.

The Discharge Summary above never states the reason for the patient's hospitalization. In fact, the author instructs readers to "See history and physical on chart"; however, that statement makes very little sense because the Discharge Summary is intended to be a stand-alone document that summarizes the patient's hospitalization. If other records are needed to support this document, then it does not fulfill its purpose or intended use. And without the history and physical, readers of this Discharge Summary do not know why the patient was hospitalized, what her complaints were, and what significant objective findings resulted in her hospitalization. Again, an aspect of The Joint Commission requirements (significant findings) are missing from the patient record shown here. Furthermore, if you recall the discussion in Chapter 7 about the importance of accurate and complete patient records, you can quickly understand how this document would not meet those expectations in any way.

Perhaps as troubling, or even more so, as the missing information is that the lab values, test results, and brief discussion are even more confusing and worrisome for readers. There is a litany of specialized tests with no explanation for why they were ordered. There are statements, like "Glucose 116. Repeated was 68," with no clarification if either or both were fasting levels or random tests. Then, in spite of the fact that one of the glucose levels appears elevated, the author states, "She had had a past history of diabetes but it certainly didn't show up on this admission." The repeated verb "had had" draws the reader's attention to the author's unrevised communication, and the lack of any medication information (at admission or during her hospitalization) further obfuscates the reader's understanding of these statements. The author's frequent writing errors add to her or his credibility issues. The sentence "Barium enema normal urogram" is completely unclear. Readers cannot be sure if the barium enema was normal or if the urogram was normal; but in either case, one of the tests does not have a result reported. And again, a breadth of seemingly unrelated, invasive, and expensive diagnostic tests are listed with no explanation for why they were ordered—especially in light of the normal results for most of them.

Finally, the conclusion of this Discharge Summary is so problematic that readers must wonder if this author is a credible provider and how capable he or she is of effectively analyzing the patient's complaints and data when the author cannot identify and correct multiple problems in this short Discharge Summary prior to signing the document. The final paragraph has multiple writing mistakes: "It was out feeling . . ." and "She recommended antacids." Clearly, the author meant "our" instead of "out." It could be argued that the transcriptionist made a mistake in transcribing the dictation, but it is not the transcriptionist's responsibility to correct incorrect verbiage. That is the author's sole responsibility, and when it does not happen, readers, especially malpractice attorneys, are left to ponder that, if an author does not use critical thinking to review and correct his or her documents, how likely is she or he to identify the patient's problems. And if the previous multiple miscues and inaccuracies were not enough, the final sentence totally befuddles the reader and makes a mockery of the author: "She will be discharged and this will be carried out." The last phrase ". . . this will be carried out" refers to the prior sentence, which states "She recommended antacids." So, it is felt that, after a vast medical workup for an unstated condition, the patient is in need of a psychiatric evaluation, but instead, the patient herself—according to the signed patient record—recommends her own treatment, and the author says "this will be carried out." It is difficult to understand how this author, based on this document, might justify this hospitalization to the patient's insurance company, but even more terrifying is how the physician–author could defend his or her care of this patient in a malpractice suit when this record serves as testament to the provider's care, communication, and critical thinking.

Let us analyze one more document before we turn our attention to authoring our own examples.

Operative Report

8/19/91

Pre-op Dx: Term pregnancy, active labor, previous Cesarean section.

Post-op Dx: Term pregnancy, active labor, previous Cesarean section.

Procedure: Low transverse Cesarean section, repeat.

Anesthesia: Spinal

Surgeons: _____, MD and _____, MD

Procedure Note:

The risks and alternatives of the procedure were explained to the patient in detail and she seems to understand. Her questions were answered. The informed consent was signed. She was taken to the Operative Suite where she was draped and prepped in the usual sterile manner. After adequate spinal anesthesia a repeat Cesarean section was performed. The incision was carried down through the old scar in the low Pfannenstiel fashion. Sharp dissection was carried down to the peritoneum. The peritoneum was tented and cut. The uterine fascia was incised in the lower uterine segment and carried bilaterally. A bladder flap was developed and a bladder blade was placed for exposure. A scalpel was utilized to make a small incision in the lower uterine segment and then the incision was carried bilaterally with the operator's fingers. The infant was suctioned and had good Apgar score. The cord was doubly clamped and cut. Cord blood was obtained. The placenta was delivered manually, single, and intact. Pitocin was added to the IV bag following delivery of the placenta. The uterus was exteriorized. The uterus was closed in three layers, fist with 0 chromic in a running interlocking fashion. Next an imbricating stitch of 0 chromic was placed with good approximation of the edges. Then the bladder flap was approximated with 000 chromic without difficulty. The gutters were cleaned of clots and the uterus was placed back in the abdomen.

Closure:

The peritoneum was closed with 000 chromic and the fascia was closed with 000 vicryl in a running fashion without difficulty. The subcutaneous tissue was closed with 000 vicryl and the skin was closed with staples. The urine was flowing and clear in the foley bag following the procedure. The patient tolerated the procedure well and there were no complications.

_____, MD

D: 8/19/91

T: 8/20/91

QUESTIONS

1. Who are the primary and secondary audiences for this particular patient record?

   Primary: _____

   _____

   _____

   Secondary: _____

   _____

   _____

2. What are the author's likely purposes for authoring this record?

   _____

   _____

   _____

   _____

3. How did the author expect this document to be used by her or his intended audience?

_____

_____

_____

4. Does anything in this record cause you confusion, or is there anything you are unclear about? If so, why?

_____

_____

_____

_____

5. Based on this document, how would you evaluate the physician–author's interactions, assessments, and decision making regarding this patient? Why?

_____

_____

_____

_____

6. Please list any necessary information that you find missing or confusing and state why.

_____

_____

_____

_____

The Operative Report shown here effectively communicates what the author did, how he or she did it, the specific results of his or her actions, and the outcome. Clearly, the audiences for this document are fairly extensive. The primary audience can be expected to include the following:

- Pediatricians caring for the neonate
- Nurses caring for the newborn
- Nurses caring for the patient
- Future healthcare providers for the patient
- Future healthcare providers for the baby
- Hospital billing personnel
- The patient's insurance company

Secondary audiences for this Operative Report are likely to be comprised of some or all of the following:

- OB–GYN residents
- Healthcare provider students
- The Joint Commission surveyors
- Malpractice attorneys

OB–GYNs, as a specialty, have the highest malpractice insurance fees nationwide. These high fees result from the high-risk nature of their work with pregnant women, especially during labor and delivery. This reality should impact more than just these specialists' insurance fees and malpractice risks. It should also affect how OB–GYNs communicate with their patients, verbally and nonverbally, and how OB–GYN–authors document those interactions and their procedures. Clearly, the purposes for the Operative Report are to describe the reason for the surgery, the type of surgery performed, the findings of the procedure, and the immediate outcome. However, as this OB–GYN–author illustrates, patient records are also an opportunity to demonstrate the provider's information sharing with the patient and to illustrate the surgeon's expertise and detail-oriented approach to health care and her or his communication effectiveness.

Clearly, it is important for the surgeon–author to have this Operative Report used as a source of information about the procedure and the specifics of what was done. However, it can also be used as documentation of the pre-operative conversation with the patient about the risks and benefits of the C-section and the fact that the patient's questions were answered and the consent form signed. By including these details in the Operative Report, the OB–GYN–author is attempting to ensure that readers can use this document to evaluate the pre-operative surgeon–patient interaction about the procedure and the patient's understanding of the risks and benefits of the operation prior to agreeing and signing the consent form. The surgeon–author wants to make it very clear that he or she personally spoke with the patient (a problem in some malpractice suits), answered the patient's questions, and obtained the patient's consent for the surgery.

However, the surgeon–author might have made this communication in the record even more clear if he or she had been as specific about the interaction as he or she was in describing the surgical procedure. For example, "she seems to understand" begs the question, Did the surgeon ask if she understood? If so, then why not document in the patient's words, "I understand." Again, the statement "Her questions were answered" might have been more helpful to readers if the author had stated what questions the patient had and how they were answered. And finally, since the consent form is supposed to be signed in the presence of the surgeon to ensure that any questions or concerns are addressed prior to the patient's signing, it would have been more clear if the OB–GYN–author had merely stated, "The informed consent was signed in my presence." As it is currently authored, "The informed consent was signed," the document still leaves open the possibility that the form was signed without the surgeon present.

Apart from these issues related to the documentation of the surgeon–author's pre-operative interaction with the patient, it would have been helpful if the record had included the infant's initial Apgar score and even the Apgar score at the end of the procedure. While these are small details, it is interesting as a reader to note the extensive specificity the surgeon–author communicates about the operative procedure. However, many of the malpractice problems for OB–GYNs related to Cesarean sections are related to the health of the infant at delivery and prior to his or her transfer to the Newborn Intensive Care Unit (NICU) or the nursery. Therefore, it would seem to be as critical for OB–GYN–authors to be as specific about the neonate's health status as it is to report in great detail about the multilayer closure.

While these two issues could clearly have been improved, it is important for providers–authors to recognize the vast amount of excellent and very effective communication in this record. One of the very critical aspects of this document that should leap out at you as you analyze it is the way that the author has organized the report. As you read it, you should be able to visualize every step in the procedure. There is no back-and-forth or confusing wording. Readers can literally follow the surgeon as she or he makes the first incision, using a well–known procedure (Pfannenstiel). Then, readers are taken through the various layers of tissue into the abdomen. The author is careful to document the small incision in "the lower uterine segment" and then to highlight that the incision is extended with "the operator's fingers" to ensure that readers know there was no risk to the fetus from the scalpel blade. And following delivery, the surgeon–author does not simply conclude with a brief discussion of his or her repair and closure. Instead, the author maintains his or her descriptive thoroughness by carefully describing each step in the postdelivery process. Finally, the author, to ensure there is no question about the patient's urinary tract and whether it had been negatively impacted by the procedure states, "the urine was flowing and clear in the foley bag following the procedure." This seemingly simple sentence documents that the bladder had not been injured during the procedure, and the patient was properly hydrated and urinating appropriately.

The author of this Operative Report demonstrates his or her understanding of many of the communication elements that we have discussed in previous chapters. It seems clear from this document that the author performed the following:

1. Utilized an authoring process
2. Analyzed the primary and secondary audiences for this document

3. Understood the purpose for the record and how it will be used
4. Recognized the importance of
   a. Complete and accurate communication
   b. Timeliness
   c. Legibility
   d. Proofreading

As discussed above, revising or re-authoring could have addressed any readers' questions regarding the infant's specific Apgar scores at delivery and at the time of transfer from the operating suite. However, in spite of those issues, this record illustrates the enormous benefits for providers–authors of analyzing each document prior to authoring it. This Operative Report stands in stark contrast to the Discharge Summary that precedes it.

If you compare the communication in the last two patient documents above, you should be able to identify a number of issues that are handled very differently by the two providers–authors. Specifically, answer the following questions related to the Discharge Summary and the Operative Report discussed above.

QUESTIONS

1. How would you compare the two documents in terms of their completeness and accuracy? Please be as specific and detailed as possible.

   _____

   _____

   _____

   _____

   _____

2. What are some of the major distinctions between the two records in terms of answering readers' questions and meeting expectations?

   _____

   _____

   _____

   _____

   _____

3. Compare the two documents in terms of their legibility. Are there issues related to one author's legible written communication versus the other (see Chapter 7)?

_____

_____

_____

_____

_____

4. How would you evaluate each author's credibility based on these two documentations of his or her medical practice?

_____

_____

_____

_____

_____

5. Which of these two records would you prefer to have authored in terms of malpractice risk, and why? Be as detailed in your explanation as possible.

_____

_____

_____

_____

_____

_____

Even though these two records have very different purposes and uses, they have several commonalities. Both are trying to communicate expected and necessary information to readers. Each record is expected to help current and future providers care for the patient who is discussed in the document. And both authors want the records to be used to demonstrate their professional acumen and credibility and to ensure that they and their organizations get reimbursed for their services. However, the differences in the communication effectiveness of the two authors are as distinct as the topics being discussed.

The Discharge Summary in this chapter is remarkable for its lack of information and for its brevity and inaccuracy. As discussed earlier, there is no information about the reason for the patient's admission, no explanation for the exhaustive and exotic tests (e.g., CT scan, lead, arsenic and mercury levels, barium enema, and urogram), and there is confusion about what the unstated final diagnosis is and what the treatment plan is going to entail. And after the breadth of normal diagnostic tests, there is the inference that it was the patient's fault that nothing was found except an ulcer and, therefore, she needed a psychiatric evaluation. Readers must question whether it was the provider's inappropriate decision making and testing or the patient's unstated psychological problem that led to all of the confusing and unexplained data in this document. However, in the end, without complete and accurate information that meets the readers' expectations and needs, it is the author who must be found responsible for this lack of communication effectiveness and obfuscation.

The differences in the two documents are also clearly illustrated by the legibility issues in the Discharge Summary in which there are uncorrected typos ("it was out feeling . . ."), unexplained inferences ("it was our feeling that possibly she should be seen in psychiatric consultation"), missing words ("Barium enema normal urogram."), and omitted data ("See history and physical on chart").

Clearly, the problems created by the ineffective information sharing in the Discharge Summary can only lead readers to question the author's professional abilities and his or her credibility as a physician. Furthermore, the lack of background and explanation and the inability of the Discharge Summary to meet The Joint Commission standards and readers' needs would likely make it a difficult document for an author to defend in a malpractice case and certainly not one she or he would be able to rely on to support his or her contentions of providing a high standard of care. These two documents are very different and highlight the potential advantages and disadvantages for authors of patient records. The problems created by and for the physician–author of the Discharge Summary are in sharp contrast to the benefits for readers and the OB–GYN–author of the Operative Report. These two documents illustrate so sharply the value for readers and authors of patient records that communicate clearly and effectively and meet readers' expectations and needs, but also, the difficulties that poorly authored and ineffective documents create for the provider–author. A patient record that does not meet the readers' needs and/or expectations is not just a communication problem, it is a potential professional liability and credibility issue for the author and his or her institution. Armed with an understanding for, and an ability to analyze, patient records, the next chapter will help you practice the authoring process and help you improve your patient documentation, health communication, and record-keeping skills.

REFERENCES

Pagano, M,. & Ragan, S. (1992). *Communication skills for professional nurses*. Newbury Park, CA: SAGE Publications.

The Joint Commission. (2009). Accreditation program: Behavioral health care 2010 Chapter: Record of care, treatment, and services. *History Tracking Report: 2010 to 2009 Requirements*, 1–20. Retrieved on October 9, 2009, from http://www.jointcommission.org/NR/rdonlyres/570CC303-8E6B-4171-ACAB-27901FE9445F/0/HistoryTracking_2010to2009_BHC_RC.pdf.

Chapter 10

Authoring Patient Records

From Start to Finish

As you begin to create various patient records, you will have the opportunity to practice authoring a wide variety of documents, or you can choose to apply the learning objectives specifically to the types of patient records you are required to author in your specific profession. As we have discussed throughout this text, the authoring process is the same regardless of the record being developed; the differences are in the format, content required and expected, and the document style. So, let us start by looking at an example of a comprehensive patient record, a History and Physical (H&P). If you have clinical opportunities, then feel free to use your actual patient's information in your record below. Otherwise, you can use the data provided in this chapter to create your revised document.

History and Physical

The H&P is a document that typically includes at a minimum some or all of the following patient information:

- Past and present complaints, illnesses, and/or injuries
- Surgeries
- Hospitalizations
- Current medications
- Allergies
- Family and social histories
- Detailed physical examination
- Preliminary or provisional diagnosi(e)s

Armed with this understanding, let us author a history based on the following patient-derived information from an emergency department (ED) visit on 3/1/2009:

Patient: Harriet Hedmaker

Present Medical History

- 45-year-old
- Caucasian female
- Lawyer
- "My stomach hurts and it's getting worse."
- 2-day history of abdominal pain.
- Pain increased with certain foods.
- Nausea, but no vomiting.
- No diarrhea.

Skills Application

1. What additional present illness information do you need to know to help guide your assessment? Be as specific and complete as possible.

   _____

   _____

   _____

   _____

   _____

2. What other information would you like to have about the patient's past medical–surgical history? Does that include the patient's allergies and current medication (if not discussed above)? Be as specific as possible.

   _____

   _____

   _____

   _____

   _____

3. Discuss the information you need to know regarding the patient's family and social histories.

_____

_____

_____

_____

_____

_____

4. What physical examination tests–findings are going to be most important to your assessment? Be as specific and complete as possible.

_____

_____

_____

_____

_____

_____

Now compare what you requested to the data provided below:

Patient: Harriet Hedmaker (Continued)

Present Medical History

Pulse = 94; blood pressure = 144/92; respirations = 16; temperature = 100.2°F (oral)

Right upper-quadrant abdominal pain, intermittently for 2 to 3 months.

No fever.

Pain increased with certain foods, especially fried foods. Spicy foods and alcohol also seem to make the pain worse.

Past Medical–Surgical History

No hospitalizations except for two vaginal deliveries of healthy children. No chronic illnesses. No surgeries. No medications. No known drug allergies. No food allergies.

Family History

Father died at 45 years of heart attack.

Mother alive at 73 years with congestive heart failure and hypertension.

Brother alive at 50 years with hypertension and hypercholesterolemia.

Sister alive at 48 years with breast cancer, treated with mastectomy and chemotherapy 4 years ago; doing well.

No knowledge about grandparents.

Social History

Currently married for past 15 years. Has a son, 8 years old, and a daughter, 11 years old, both in good health. Personal injury attorney for 19 years. Sexually active; denies multiple partners; denies STDs; uses condoms for birth control. Last menstrual period 3 weeks ago.

Drinks 2 to 3 glasses of wine three to four times per week. Denies any other drug use.

Review of Systems

Negative except for above.

Physical Examination Findings

Negative except for the following positive observations:

5'4" female weighing 168 pounds.

Abdomen = soft, tender in right upper quadrant, with positive Murphy's sign.

Based on the information provided here, or based on your own clinical experience with a specific patient, please answer the following questions in as much detail as possible:

Skills Application

1. Who would you include as the likely primary and secondary audiences for this patient record (H&P)?

Primary: _____

_____

_____

Secondary: _____

_____

_____

_____

2. What are your major purposes for authoring this record? Be as detailed as possible.

_____

_____

_____

_____

3. Discuss in detail, how you expect your primary and secondary readers to use this document, based on your patient's complaints, your findings, and your preliminary diagnosis? Be as specific and detailed as possible.

_____

_____

_____

_____

4. In the space below, create an H&P based on the information you collected from your clinical experience or from the information supplied above. Be sure to provide a preliminary–working diagnosis–assessment and a treatment plan.

_____

_____

_____

_____

_____

_____

_____

_____

_____

History and Physical

Patient's Name: _____   **Provider's Name:** _____

Date: _____

Chief Complaint: _____

_____

Present Medical History: _____

_____

_____

_____

_____

_____

Past Medical History: _____

_____

_____

_____

_____

Family History: _____

_____

_____

_____

_____

Social History: _____

_____

_____

_____

Review of Systems: _____

_____

_____

_____

_____

Physical Examination

Vital Signs: pulse _____; respirations ___/___; blood pressure _____;
temperature _____ F

General: _____

_____

HEENT: _____

_____

_____

Neck: _____

Chest: _____

Heart: _____

Abdomen: _____

_____

_____

Genital/Rectal: _____

_____

_____

Neurologic: _____

_____

_____

Musculoskeletal: _____

Preliminary Diagnosis: _____

_____

Treatment Plan: _____

_____

_____

Signature: _____

Now that you have done your pre-authoring assessment of the audience, purpose, and use for this document, as well as determined the critical content to provide based on that analysis, and written the record, you are ready to review–revise the document by going back and examining how your authored draft above meets, exceeds, or falls short of your pre-authoring analysis. Be sure to revise (add, change, or delete) any areas that do not fulfill your audience, purpose, and use analysis. Remember to make any changes to this document using the proofreading changes described in Chapters 6 and 7. Now, let us look at how you might have completed this H&P if you used the data supplied above.

History and Physical

Patient's Name: Harriet Hedmaker   **Provider's Name:** _____

Date: 3/1/2009

Chief Complaint: "My stomach hurts and it's getting worse."

Present Medical History: 45-year-old, Caucasian female, with a 2–3 month history of intermittent right upper quadrant abdominal pain. Pain has increased over the last 2 days, "8/10" per patient today in the ED. She denies fever, but "I haven't taken it." She denies vomiting, diarrhea, hematemesis, melena, or hematochezia; however, she does complain of nausea. She states that "spicy foods and alcohol make it worse and fried foods are really bad." She denies any similar symptoms prior to first noticing them 2–3 months ago. Her last menstrual period was 2/8/2009 and was normal for flow, duration, and timing.

Past Medical History: The patient denies having any surgeries or chronic illnesses. She was hospitalized only twice, both times for a vaginal delivery of healthy children. She is on no medications and denies any food or drug allergies.

Family History: She has no knowledge of her fraternal or maternal grandparents, "They were dead before I was born." Her father died of a myocardial infarction at age 45. Her mother is alive at 73 and lives independently, but has hypertension and congestive heart failure. The patient has one brother, age 50 with hypertension and hypercholesterolemia. Her only sister is 48 and alive and a breast cancer survivor with a mastectomy and chemotherapy in 2005. She has a healthy son aged 8 and a healthy daughter aged 11.

Social History: The patient is married for 15 years, no divorces. She is a personal injury lawyer for the past 19 years. She is sexually active, denies multiple partners or sexually transmitted diseases, and uses condoms for birth control. She drinks "2–3 glasses of wine 3–4 days per week." She denies any recreational drug usage. Her husband is a police officer.

Review of Systems: HEENT: No hair loss, headaches, or scalp lesions; no ear pain, or hearing loss, no eye pain, visual changes, or diplopia; no sinus pain, frequent URIs, or sinusitis; no nose bleeds or nasal congestion; no sore throat, dental problems, oral lesions, or dysphagia. Neck: no pain with range of motion or lymph node enlargement; Chest: no pain, no shortness of breath, no cough, no dyspnea; Heart: no tachycardia; no chest, neck, or left arm pain, no high blood pressure, no paroxysmal nocturnal dyspnea, and she has

1 pillow orthopnea: Abdomen: frequent flatulence, otherwise, pain and symptoms as discussed above; GU/Rectal: denies vaginal or rectal bleeding, no vaginal discharge, no dyspareunia, no hemorrhoids or changes in bowel movements—usually every other day and same size and consistency; Neurologic; no vertigo, no memory loss, no tremors; Musculoskeletal: no weakness in extremities, no ataxia, no rashes, no lesions, no gait changes.

Physical Examination

Vital Signs: pulse 94; respirations 16; blood pressure 144 /92; temperature 100.2°F. (oral)

General: Well-developed, well-nourished, overweight, 45-year-old white female in mild distress at the time of this examination. Pain level "8/10."

HEENT: Normal cephalic, no scalp lesions. Ear canals are clear, TMs reflective, EOMs are intact, PERRLA, fundi show sharp disc margins bilaterally without hemorrhages or exudates. Sinuses are nontender bilaterally, nares are patent. Mouth and pharynx have no lesions, no erythema, and no dental caries.

Neck: Supple with full ROM, no anterior or posterior lymphadenopathy.

Chest: Clear to auscultation, no rales, rhonchi, or wheezes. Normal diaphragmatic excursion

Heart: Regular rate and rhythm without murmurs. Carotid pulses are equal bilaterally and free of bruits. Peripheral pulses are 2+ and equal—brachial, radial, inguinal, and pedal.

Abdomen: Soft, tender, right upper-quadrant with positive Murphy's sign. Some guarding in the RUQ, but no rebound tenderness. Bowel sounds normal-active, no guarding, tenderness or rebound anywhere else in the abdomen. Palpation = liver edge 2 fingerbreadths distal to right anterior costal margin. Spleen is not palpable. No masses are palpated, no abdominal bruits.

Genital/Rectal: Vaginal exam shows no cervical motion tenderness, no discharge, and no adnexal masses. No ovarian or uterine masses or enlargement. Rectal = normal sphincter tone, no masses, brown stool, GUAIAC negative.

Neurologic: Alert and oriented to time, place, and person. Cranial nerves II through XII intact. Reflexes 2+ and = upper and lower extremities bilaterally. Babinski negative.

Musculoskeletal: Full ROM in all joint, no pain with ROM. No rashes or lesions.

Preliminary Diagnosis:

1. Probable cholecystitis
2. Rule out cholelithiasis
3. Rule out duodenal or peptic ulcer

Treatment Plan: NPO, IV fluids, admission, Ultrasound of gallbladder, pain medication prn; surgical and/or gastroenterologist consult.

Signature: _____

Compare this example to your pre-writing analysis.

Skills Application

1. Does this record address the primary and secondary readers' expectations and needs? If so, why and how? If no, why not?

_____

_____

_____

_____

2. Does this example meet the multiple purposes you identified? If yes, why and how? If no, why not?

_____

_____

_____

3. Can this example be used as intended in your prewriting analysis? If yes, why and how? If no, why not?

_____

_____

_____

4. Does the content supplied in this example meet your expectations and needs? If so, why? If not, what is missing, unclear, or inaccurate?

_____

_____

_____

_____

As you evaluated this example, you should have asked yourself if readers could obtain the information they needed to assess the patient's complaints, the provider's findings, and the treatment plans and decisions. Both primary and secondary readers will want to evaluate not just the content but the breadth of information obtained as well (from the patient's narrative and the provider-patient interaction, as well as from the provider's examination). Readers will expect to use the details—qualitative and quantitative, subjective and objective—to help them assess the provider's critical thinking and decision making.

As we have discussed throughout this text, the ability of readers to accurately and sufficiently gather needed data depends entirely on the author's communication effectiveness in the patient record. While you may feel there are specific items or pieces of information that are not contained in this example, the key question remains, does this record fulfill what you determined were its purposes, for the intended audiences, and expected uses?

Now, let us turn our attention to a different record and continue our pre-authoring and revising analyses, as well as practicing our written communication skills.

Nurse's Note

Here is some important information for you to use in creating your Nurse's Note. As we mentioned previously, if you have a clinical opportunity to gather information from a patient, feel free to use that data instead of what is presented here.

Patient: Ms. Lotus

Setting: A 20-year-old woman was admitted to the Labor Room at 1840 hours [10/2/2008]. Nurse Heidi Colb (fictitious name) did an assessment, checked her fetal heart tones, evaluated her degree of dilatation and reported her findings to Dr. Henry Jameson, the obstetrician who is on call for the patient's doctor, Martha Goode. By 2200 hours the patient is dilated 6 centimeters and requesting an epidural anesthetic.

Ms. Lotus: "I need an epidural, I can't take any more of this pain."

Nurse Colb: "I've called Dr. Bijou, the anesthesiologist who's on call tonight, and he'll be here in just a couple of minutes"

Ms. Lotus: "Oh my God, it hurts so bad!"

With that statement the patient suddenly rolled over, slammed against the plastic side rail, which snapped into pieces, and the patient tumbled onto the floor. She did not lose consciousness. The Nurse Colb pressed the emergency call button to summon help without leaving the patient's side. She questioned the patient about any areas of pain and assessed the patient quickly. Once help arrived, she got her back into bed. Following the incident, the patient's fetal heart tones, as well as the record on the fetal monitor, were unchanged [from prior to the fall]. Nurse Colb notified Dr. Jameson of the patient's fall and her assessment.

The patient's labor progressed rapidly, and at 2300 hours the patient was taken to the Delivery Room and gave birth to a 9-pound 2-ounce boy. Both mother and baby were doing fine as Heidi Colb sat at the nurses' desk and began to consider how she was going to document the patient's fall, her assessment, interventions, communication of the event, and the patient's response to the accident. (Pagano & Ragan, 1992, pp. 103–104)

This example is specific to nursing; however, as you should recognize, a similar type of incident could have occurred in a wide variety of settings with any healthcare provider. As you should realize, taking care of the patient is your first priority; however, once you have accomplished that goal and notified the necessary parties, how you document in the patient record what happened, what you did, and what you determined will go a long way in determining how the incident is evaluated in the weeks, months, and years ahead—especially if it leads to litigation against your institution and/or yourself. For the purpose of this exercise, you need to see yourself as Nurse Colb (again it is the communication that is important here, so try not to let the profession obfuscate your learning). As Nurse Colb, please complete the pre-authoring assessment below for this incident.

Skills Application

1. What information do you need to provide to your audience about this event? Be as specific and as complete as possible.

_____

_____

_____

_____

_____

_____

2. Who are the likely primary and secondary audiences for this patient record? Be specific.

   Primary: _____

   _____

   _____

   Secondary: _____

   _____

   _____

3. What are the purposes for this document, and how might they be altered by the incident?

   _____

   _____

   _____

   _____

   _____

   _____

   _____

4. How do you want your primary and secondary readers to use this document, and how is that different than it would be if there were not an incident?

   _____

   _____

   _____

   _____

   _____

   _____

   _____

Based on your pre-authoring analyses and the content supplied above, please create a Nurse's Note for the time frame 2200 hours until the mother and baby were returned to the room at 2335 hours. Try not to dwell on the fact that this is a Nurse's Note, but instead concentrate on being an author whose role is to communicate information to primary and secondary readers to meet or exceed their expectations and needs and to fulfill your purposes and the intended uses for this document. Concentrate on communicating effectively and recognize the universality of the assignment for any healthcare provider.

Nurse's Note

2200 hrs.: _____

_____

_____

_____

_____

_____

_____

_____

_____

_____

_____

_____

_____

_____

_____

_____

_____

_____

_____

_____

_____

_____

_____

_____

As you authored this record, how did you feel about the experience?

QUESTIONS

1. Was it difficult to determine how much information to include in the record? If yes, why? If no, why not?

2. Did you recall what you learned in Chapter 7 about completeness and thoroughness? If so, how did that help you decide what to include? If not, do you think it might have helped if you had considered it, and why or why not?

3. What content did you feel was most important for you to highlight and why? Please be specific and detailed.

Let us look at the actual patient record, previously discussed in Chapter 3, of how a nurse–author documented the information about Ms. Lotus and the incident described above.

Nurse's Note

2200 hrs.:   Patient had a contriction [*sic*] and rolled around on the bed until she fell to the floor. She didn't lose consciousness and she didn't complain of any pain, except in her gluteal area.

2230 hrs.:   Dr. Jameson and Dr. Bijou in to see patient. Epidural anesthetic given. Patient's vital signs and fetal heart tone are ok.

2255 hrs.:   Fully dilated moved to Delivery.

2311 hrs.:   Vaginal delivery of 9.2 pound boy with APGAR [sic] of 9.

2335 hrs.:   Mother and baby returned to Room 512. (Pagano & Ragan, 1992, p. 107)

Skills Application

1. How does this patient record meet your expectations and needs as a reader based on your pre-authoring analysis for this document?

_____

_____

_____

_____

2. Based on the Chapter 7, what problems can you identify in this patient record? Be as specific and detailed as possible.

_____

_____

_____

_____

_____

_____

3. What specific content do you think could have been added and/or revised to enhance the communication effectiveness of this patient record? Why?

_____

_____

_____

_____

4. Compare this nurse–author's documentation with the record you created above. How do the two compare? From a reader's perspective, what are

the strengths and weaknesses of each, and which one do you think is more effective, and why?

_____

_____

_____

_____

_____

_____

_____

_____

Now that you have evaluated these two attempts at communicating the incident and surrounding events, let us examine another alternative.

Nurse's Note

10/2/08

2200 hrs.: Ms. Lotus was having contractions about 2 minutes apart. The fetal heart rate was 148. The patient had an apparent contraction, and, while screaming in pain she rolled abruptly onto her left side and struck the side rail that was raised to prevent her from rolling off the bed. However, the left side rail broke and the patient rolled about 2 feet from the bed to the floor. She landed on her gluteal area and did not strike her head or her abdomen. I was standing a few feet from the patient dialing Dr. Jameson to tell him that Dr. Bijou was coming up to start the epidural when the patient screamed and tumbled to the floor. She had no loss of consciousness. I asked Ms. Lotus if she hurt anywhere and she replied, "my butt is a little sore, but that's all."

2205 hrs.: After pressing the emergency buzzer, I made the patient rest on the floor until nurses Mary Beth O'Connor and Billie May Britton arrived to help get the patient into a new bed with intact side rails. While the other nurses checked the patient's vital signs, I used the Doppler and checked the fetal heart rate that was 149. Ms. Lotus's pulse before the fall had been 92 and it was still 92 afterward, her blood pressure was unchanged at 124/80, and her respirations had increased slightly from 20 before the fall to 24 afterward. She had clear breath sounds throughout both lungs. I then notified Dr. Jameson about the incident and Ms. Lotus's vital signs, fetal heart rate, and that she was alert and well-oriented and not complaining of any pain except her labor, which continued with hard contractions 2 minutes apart. Dr. Jameson did not give any new orders. I then notified Celia Horn, the Labor Room Supervisor, about the patient's fall and her condition.

2220 hrs.: The patient's breath sounds remain clear, her heart rate is regular and unchanged. Her abdomen is soft, except during her contractions, and she had normal active bowel sounds and no abdominal tenderness except with her contractions.

2230 hrs.: Dr. Jameson arrived and examined the patient who denied any complaints except her labor. Dr. Bijou administered the epidural.

2245 hrs.: Ms. Lotus states, "I'm much better, that was good stuff he put in there."

2255 hrs.: Dr. Jameson notified that the patient is completely dilated and fully effaced. Patient transferred to the Delivery Room.

2311 hrs.: Patient had a vaginal delivery of a 9 lb., 2 oz. boy without difficulty. APGAR was 9.

2335 hrs.: Ms. Lotus and her baby out of the Delivery Room without any problems and returned to Room 512 for rooming-in. The infant's APGAR was 10 when taken from the Delivery Room.

Heidi Colb, RN

Skills Application

1. How does this alternative patient record meet your expectations and needs as a reader based on your pre-authoring analysis for this document?

_____

_____

_____

_____

2. Based on the Chapter 7, what problems can you identify in this patient record compared to the original? Be as specific and detailed as possible.

_____

_____

_____

_____

_____

_____

3. What specific content do you think could have been added and/or revised to enhance the communication effectiveness of this patient record? Why?

_____

_____

_____

_____

_____

4. Compare this documentation with the earlier record and the one you created above. How do the three compare? From a reader's perspective, what are the strengths and weaknesses of each, and which one do you think is more effective, and why?

_____

_____

_____

_____

_____

_____

_____

_____

As you examined each of the records, were you able to identify the ways in which an author can communicate information that makes him or her appear more credible and professional without changing the details–content? Hopefully, you were able to see how the alternative Nurse's Note was able to meet or exceed the readers' expectations and needs for thoroughness and completeness. For example, the original Nurse's Note does not mention that the bedrails were up—only that the patient fell out of bed. How difficult do you think it would be for Nurse Colb, 2 or 3 years later in a deposition or at trial, to recall if the fall described in the original Nurse's Note occurred with the rails up or down? This need for specificity is at the heart of what we are discussing and practicing in this chapter.

Is this level of documentation necessary for uncomplicated deliveries? Probably not, but the context for this patient record is certainly not typical or ordinary. A patient fall is certainly a risk to the patient, but frequently a legal risk for the provider and the institution. However, when the patient is pregnant, the risks are obviously increased for everyone, and how the information about the incident is communicated will likely go a long way to determining the hospital's liability and, in this case, the nurse–author's culpability and professionalism.

You likely noted the spelling errors in the first example. How would you think those errors might impact any legal issues related to this case? If you were the plaintiff–patient's attorney or a juror, would you question the professionalism and credibility of a nurse–author who cannot spell or proofread the document she or he created? And if you find the nurse–author less credible and professional for spelling mistakes, how might that lead to your perception of his or her skills as a nurse, as a documenter of what actually occurred in that room, and so forth? The problem for healthcare providers is that when their documents do not meet readers' expectations and needs, especially when they are incomplete, illegible, and/or inaccurate, the provider–author's professional qualifications, legitimacy, and credibility may suffer.

Let us look at some of the specific strategies used in the alternative record. For example, the nurse–author is much more complete and thorough in the alternate record. In addition, the author uses quotes from the patient to make the document less subjective and more detailed. It is one thing for a provider–author to state in a record that the patient only had pain in her gluteal area, but it is far more persuasive to readers if the author reports the patient's own words, "My butt is a little sore, but that's all." By doing this, the author takes away the reader's questions or concerns about what was said and what was translated by the provider. In quoting the patient, all readers can equally assess the patient's evaluation of the location and quantification of the postincident pain. In addition, the alternate record has far more objective data and includes pulse, respirations, blood pressure, and fetal heart tones both pre- and postincident. And readers are told not just the baby's postdelivery Apgar score, but the Apgar score when he left the delivery room.

It seems obvious that this nurse used a pre-authoring analysis to evaluate the situation and the potential primary and secondary readers' questions and/or concerns. By avoiding gaps in the record and documenting who was present and when for each step in the postincident and delivery process, the audience can not only follow along as the patient is being cared for but can be expected to find the author more credible and professional and less likely to be responsible in any way for the event. This persuasion, through careful and thorough documentation as discussed in Chapter 7, is an ideal way for providers to communicate information and to ensure that readers perceive the author as a credible healthcare professional.

Based on your learnings to this point, let us move on to a different example and a different type of patient record. Examine the following to see what impact you think the format and recording style have on a patient document.

The following record is verbatim (including all abbreviations) and was hand-written in the original (italicized in this version = handwritten in original).

History and Physical

Chief Complaint: *Intestinal obstruction.*

Present Illness: *41 y.o. F, RN with 6 d hx of nausea, emesis, abd tenderness. Was seen in ER 4 d ago & felt to be slightly dehydrated, rx-ed with IV fluid. Sx's started after eating seafood. No hematemesis, melena. Today Sx's worsening-pain ≠ but still not very severe; feels she is dehydrated. X-ray today shows dilated; edematous loops s. bowel but air in rectum.*

Past History: *10 y ago–R oophorectomy & cyst removal*

Social History: *RN, Single*

Family History: *N/C*

Current and/or Recently Used Medications: *Phenergan*

Allergies (drugs or anesthesia): *None*

Review of Systems: *Current illness only*

Report of Physical Examination:

Vital Signs: *BP. 110/70 T. 99 P. 80 R. 16*

General Appearance, Mental Status: *WDWF in NAD, cooperative*

Check Appropriate Column.

	No Abnormalities Noted	See Comments	Comments–Abnormal Findings
Skin:	*X*		
Lymphatics:	*X*		
HEENT:	*X*		
Neck:	*X*		
Breasts:	*X*		
Chest and Lungs:	*X*		

Heart–Size:			
Rhythm:			
Murmurs:			*holosyst at LSB & Apex*
Vascular:	*X*		
Abdomen:		*X*	*hi pitched bowel snds; Moderate distention*
Genitalia:			*deferred (LMP 1 week)*
Rectal:	*X*		
Extremities:	*X*		
Neurological:	*X*		

Provisional Diagnosis: *Intestinal Obstruction—Partial Small Bowel.*

_____, MD

Skills Application

1. How would you evaluate, as a primary or secondary reader, the H&P above? Please be as specific as you can be in your assessment.

   _____

   _____

   _____

   _____

   _____

   _____

2. Based on the information provided, what do you know specifically about the patient's rectal exam? Be as detailed as possible.

   _____

   _____

   _____

3. How would you compare the information presented in this handwritten checklist to information provided in a computerized checklist? What is your opinion as an author of patient records and a reader of this format? Why?

   _____

   _____

_____

_____

_____

4. What specific history and physical information does the patient record above not provide that you expect or need to assess this patient's problem and the provider–author's care? Be as specific and detailed as possible.

_____

_____

_____

_____

_____

_____

_____

Please use the information provided and any additional information that you feel is needed to create an H&P that fulfills the intended audiences' needs and expectations; is complete, thorough, and legible; and addresses the purposes and uses for this particular patient document. Be as detailed in your authoring as possible and create whatever information you feel is lacking in the original to make your H&P communicate effectively.

History and Physical

Chief Complaint: _____

Present Illness: _____

_____

_____

_____

_____

Past History: _____

_____

_____

_____

Social History: _____

_____

_____

_____

Family History: _____

_____

_____

_____

Current and/or Recently Used Medications: Phenergan

Allergies (drugs or anesthesia): None

Review of Systems: _____

_____

_____

_____

_____

_____

_____

Report of Physical Examination:

Vital Signs: <u>BP. 110/70 T. 99 P. 80 R. 16</u>

General Appearance, Mental Status: _____

_____

Skin: _____

_____

_____

Lymphatics: _____

_____

HEENT: _____

_____

Neck: _____

_____

Breasts: _____

_____

Chest and Lungs: _____

_____

_____

_____

Heart–Size: _____

_____

_____

_____

Vascular: _____

_____

Abdomen: _____

_____

_____

_____

_____

_____

Genitalia: _____

_____

Rectal: _____

_____

Extremities: _____

_____

Neurological: _____

_____

_____

_____

Provisional Diagnosis: _____

_____

_____

_____

Skills Application

1. What information, in general, did you think was critical to detail in your H&P that was missing from the original? Why?

   _____

   _____

   _____

   _____

   _____

2. How did your Provisional Diagnosis differ from the original? Why?

   _____

   _____

   _____

   _____

3. Did you change any of the abbreviations from the original? If so, which ones, and why? If no, why not?

   _____

   _____

   _____

   _____

4. How and why do you think your revised H&P better addresses the purposes and uses for this patient record than the original? Please be as specific and detailed as possible.

   _____

   _____

   _____

   _____

The original patient record illustrates many of the problems addressed throughout this book. As authored, it is unclear, incomplete, illegible (for example handwritten and abbreviations), and not thorough in many areas. It does not take into account the audiences' needs or expectations, and it does not fulfill the most basic purposes and uses for an H&P: information sharing, effective communication, and demonstration of logical decision making.

The provider–author tells readers in the Chief Complaint "intestinal obstruction," yet the Chief Complaint is expected to be the patient's subjective statement about her problem. However, it seems highly doubtful that this was her stated chief complaint. In fact, the provider author records in the Present Illness, ". . . feels she is dehydrated" (not in quotes in the original). This subjective statement from the patient would seem to be her chief complaint; however, readers have no way of assessing it based on this document. In fact, the provider–author mentions dehydration twice in the Present Illness section, yet never refers to it again anywhere in the record. Therefore, readers are unable to determine if she is dehydrated.

This confusion about her possible dehydration could have been easily rectified by a physical examination that described her oral mucosa, skin turgor, and urine-specific gravity and/or BUN and creatinine levels. However, the provider fails to recognize, because of a clear lack of pre-authoring analysis, the importance of this information for the reader. Perhaps even more critical for readers is the lack of specific physical examination findings related to the patient's abdominal, vaginal, and rectal exams. This missing specific information ("No abnormalities noted") is compounded by the provider–author's statement that he or she "deferred" a pelvic exam in a patient with abdominal pain. Therefore, readers have no way to be certain that there is not a pelvic mass that is responsible for the patient's ileus, pain, and partial obstruction.

Finally, the brief Provisional Diagnosis leaves readers wondering how thorough, complete, and credible this provider–author is in his or her evaluations and decision making if he or she only lists "Intestinal Obstruction— Partial Small Bowel" as the possible assessment. For example, would the provider not want to mention the possibility of a tumor or adhesions from previous surgery as potential causes for the obstruction? And as discussed in the previous paragraph, what about an ectopic pregnancy, appendicitis, or even diverticulitis as potential etiologies? The lack of information in this H&P, especially as it relates to the expected audiences' questions about the specifics of the provider's abdominal, vaginal, and rectal exams, is a major problem for the author. That issue, coupled with the brief and poorly communicated initial assessment, contributes to readers' likely concerns about the provider's professional skills, critical thinking, and credibility as a healthcare professional.

Here is an example of how the original H&P might have been created using the pre-authoring process and the information learned in Chapter 7 and in the other chapters of this text.

History and Physical

Chief Complaint: <u>"My stomach hurts and I feel dehydrated."</u>

Present Illness: <u>41-year-old female who has a 6-day history of nausea, vomiting, and upper abdominal tenderness. Her symptoms started after eating seafood. She denies any hematemesis, melena, or hematochezia. Her last bowel movement was 2 days prior to this admission. She was seen in the ED 4 days ago for similar symptoms, felt to be dehydrated and given IV fluids. Today she complains of worsening pain, rated by her at "6/10." However, she is concerned that she may be dehydrated from her frequent vomiting, 5–10 times/day yesterday and today. She's unable to keep anything down, in spite of the Phenergan suppositories she was prescribed on discharge from the ED. A flat and upright abdominal x-ray today reveals dilated loops of small bowel, however, air is visible in the rectum. Her urine specific gravity is 1.035 and her BUN is 22 with a creatinine of 2.2.</u>

Past History: <u>No chronic illnesses, no daily medications, except Phenergan suppositories started 4 days ago prn nausea/vomiting on discharge from ED. Gravida 2, Para. 2, Aborta 0. Both children were products of uncomplicated vaginal deliveries. Surgeries: R. oophorectomy & cyst removal in 1999.</u>

Social History: <u>Registered Nurse, married, with two sons. She denies smoking or recreational drug use. She has "a couple of glasses of wine a week." She exercises at the hospital's gym for 20–30 minutes, 3–4 times/week. She is sexually active, monogamous, and uses condoms for birth control.</u>

Family History: <u>Father died at age 63 of an MI; mother is alive at age 70 with breast and uterine cancer. Patient is an only child and she's unsure of what her grandparents died from. Her husband and sons are in good health.</u>

Current and/or Recently Used Medications: <u>Phenergan</u>

Allergies (drugs or anesthesia): <u>None Known Drug Allergies</u>

Review of Systems: <u>General: no major change in weight, prior to this illness, no sleep difficulties. Skin: no rashes, lesions, or changes in nevi. HEENT: no ear pain, decrease in hearing, no change in visual acuity, does not wear glasses or contacts, no diplopia, no sinus pain or nasal discharge, no epistaxsis, no dental caries, oral lesions, or dysphagia. Neck: no pain.</u>

Chest: no shortness of breath, cough, or sputum production. Heart: no chest pain, paroxysmal nocturnal dyspnea, no orthopnea (sleeps on one pillow), no pedal edema, murmur since childhood. Abdomen: no vomiting, nausea, reflux, ulcers, or diarrhea. No food intolerances. No hematemesis, hematochezia, or melena. No prior colonoscopy. GYN: regular menstrual periods, last one was 1 week ago, normal timing, length, and quantity. No discharge, odor, or dyspareunia. Rectal: No hemorrhoids, no change in bowel consistency, size, or volume prior to this illness. Musculoskeletal: no pain in joints or muscles, no difficulty with range of motion, no weakness, no back or neck complaints. Neurological: no vertigo, tremors, or paresthesias.

Report of Physical Examination:

Vital Signs: BP. 110/70 T. 99 P. 80 R. 16

General Appearance, Mental Status: Well-developed, well-nourished, ill-appearing 41-year-old Caucasian female who is in some distress at the time of this examination. She is alert and oriented to time, place, and person.

Skin: Warm, dry, but with decreased skin turgor and slowed capillary refill.

Lymphatics: No palpable or enlarged cervical, axillary, or inguinal lymph nodes.

HEENT: Normal cephalic, hair normal texture and distribution, no scalp lesions, Ears: canals clear bilaterally with reflective TMs. Eyes: EOMs intact, PERRLA, fundoscopic exam = sharp disk margins bilaterally without hemorrhages or exudates. Nose: patent, sinuses nontender. Throat: no dental caries, no oral lesions, and no erythema.

Neck: Carotids are equal bilaterally and free of bruits. Full ROM without pain, thyroid is symmetrical, without nodules or enlargement.

Breasts: Symmetrical, no masses, no discharge.

Chest and Lungs: Clear to auscultation and percussion bilaterally, no rales, rhonchi, or wheezes. Normal diaphragmatic excursion.

Heart–Size: Regular rate and rhythm with a grade 2/6 holosystolic murmur heard best at the left sternal border and apex (present since childhood per patient).

Vascular: Carotid, radial, brachial, inguinal, and posterior tibial pulses 2+ and equal bilaterally. No abdominal or carotid bruits.

Abdomen: Distended, firm, with high-pitched bowel sounds, no tinkles or rushes. No masses are palpated; liver and spleen edges cannot be palpated secondary to distention. Increased tenderness in right upper and lower quadrant with guarding, but no rebound. Left abdomen nontender.

Genitalia: Vaginal exam reveals no discharge, or odor, no external or internal lesions. There is no cervical motion tenderness. There is a fullness in the right adnexa with tenderness, but no mass could be palpated. Left adnexa nontender.

Rectal: Normal sphincter tone, no masses or tenderness, no stool. Guaiac negative.

Extremities: Full ROM in both upper and lower extremities. No weakness in upper or lower extremities, right versus left. No edema, no masses.

Neurological: Alert and oriented x3, cranial nerves II through XII intact. Reflexes 2+ and equal in upper and lower extremities bilaterally. Babinski negative bilaterally.

Provisional Diagnosis:

1. Small bowel obstruction
2. Dehydration
3. Appendicitis vs. adhesions
4. Rule out right-sided abdominal mass

Now that you have written your alternate H&P and read the one above, take a minute to compare both of these to the original and then answer the questions below.

Skills Application

1. How does your rewrite and the alternate above compare to the original in terms of audience expectations and the intended purposes and uses for the document? Please be specific.

_____

_____

_____

_____

_____

2. In what ways do you think the information communicated in your revision and the one above alter your assessment of the Provisional Diagnosis? How about your assessment of the provider–author?

_____

_____

_____

_____

_____

3. How did the narrative format, as compared to the checklist, impact your perceptions and analysis of the author's exam and critical thinking? Please be as specific as possible.

    _____

    _____

    _____

    _____

4. In what ways do you think the fact that the original document was hand-written, versus the printed alternate above, impact the author's communication effectiveness in each? Why?

    _____

    _____

    _____

    _____

The alternate H&P shown above and hopefully in the one you authored strive to communicate thorough, clear, and expected information to the likely primary and secondary audiences for this record. The importance of using the authoring process to analyze the audience, purpose, and use for each patient record and then reviewing and proofreading to ensure that the document accomplishes your goals and objectives should be more obvious as you explore these records, your analyses of them, and your own rewrites and the alternates presented above.

Let us examine one final example to continue expanding our appreciation for the authoring process and the value of thoughtful analysis.

Physical Therapy Note

Date: 1/3/09

Referred by: Dr. _____ with a diagnosis of KNEE STRAIN (L)

Age/Sex: 32/F

Precautions:

Insurance: W/COMP

Visit Note: RE-EVALUATION

S: LAT KNEE PAIN AND STILL PAIN ON LOW BACK

O: PATELLAR MOB

STRETCHING HIP FLEXORS/HAMSTRING

A: L ELEVATED IC CORRECTED AFTER SESSON; WILL SEE DR. _____

ON MONDAY. NOW + TENDERNESS IN R TIOBIO-FIBULAR AREA

NOW–TENDERNESS ON INFERIOR PATELLAR BURSA

KNEE ROM = WFL

MMT

HIP FLEXORS = 4

KNEE EXTENSORS = 4

NEW STG IN 4 WEEKS:

1. INC STRENGTH ON L LE

2. INDEP HEP

P: CONT POC 1-2XWK 4WKS FOR LE STRENGTHENING. WILL CONT

THERAPY FOR CORE AND STABILIZATION EX

PLEASE SIGN BELOW IF AGREEABLE TO PLAN OF CARE AND RETURN BY

FAX. THANK YOU VERY MUCH!!

X _____   DR. _____

X _____   _____, PT

Skills Application

1. As you read the note above, what information did you find helpful? Was any of it troubling or confusing? Why?

_____

_____

_____

_____

_____

2. How would you evaluate this provider–author based on the realization that this record is not intended for an orthopedic surgeon? Please explain your answer.

_____

_____

_____

_____

_____

3. How did the Subjective, Objective, Assessment, Plan (SOAP) Note format impact your perceptions and analysis of the authors' exam, treatment, assessments, and plans? Please be as specific as possible.

_____

_____

_____

_____

4. What would you change in this document to make it better meet the purposes and uses it is intended for? Why?

_____

_____

_____

_____

5. Did the use of lowercase initially and then uppercase cause you any concerns? If so, why? If no, why not?

_____

_____

_____

_____

It may interest you to know that numerous providers in occupational health clinics were shown this record, and none of them knew what all the abbreviations meant. And this record was authored for occupational health providers.

In order for you to revise this document you will likely need to know what these abbreviations in the original record stand for:

ROM = range of motion
MOB = mobility
IC = iliac crest
HEP = home exercise program
MMT = manual muscle testing
WFL = within functional limits
STG = staging
W/COMP = workers' compensation

Armed with this information, please rewrite the note above and try to make it meet your analysis of the audience (primary and secondary), purpose(s), and uses for this document. Strive to be as complete, clear, legible, and thorough as possible.

Physical Therapy Note

Date: 1/3/09

Referred by: Dr.   with a diagnosis of

Age/Sex: 32/F

Precautions:

Insurance: W/COMP

Visit Note: RE-EVALUATION

   S:

   O:

   A:

   P:

_____

_____

PLEASE SIGN BELOW IF AGREEABLE TO PLAN OF CARE AND RETURN BY FAX.
THANK YOU VERY MUCH

X _____   DR. _____

X _____   _____, PT

QUESTIONS

1. As you revised the note above, how did you determine what information was important for the primary and secondary audiences? Why?

   _____

   _____

   _____

   _____

   _____

2. What decisions as the provider–author of your revised document did you make regarding the use of all caps and abbreviations? Why?

   _____

   _____

   _____

   _____

   _____

3. Did you find the SOAP Note format provided you with an opportunity to communicate effectively with your audience and for your intended purposes and uses? Why, or why not?

   _____

   _____

   _____

   _____

4. How is the author's credibility impacted by the communication in the original record versus your revised document? Why?

   _____

   _____

_____

_____

5. Based on the discussions of legibility in Chapter 7, how did your revised
   document meet the standards described in that chapter? Do you feel that
   legibility was an important issue in the original versus your revised
   record? Why, or why not?

_____

_____

_____

_____

Clearly, the original note above created many problems for the record's
intended audiences. While it might be argued that orthopedic surgeons, with
their frequent use of physical therapy for their patients, could be expected to
know the vast number of abbreviations used in this document, the same would
not be true for the majority of the other primary and secondary audiences:

Primary
- Occupational medicine providers
- Workers' compensation case managers
- Primary care providers

Secondary
- Healthcare provider students
- Malpractice–workers' compensation attorneys

If one of the major purposes for any patient record is the communication of
information needed to care for the patient, then the original Patient Note above
clearly fails to meet that goal. And if the provider–author of the original note
expected it to be used as an illustration of her or his professional abilities and
credibility as a provider, it would seem unlikely that it would be used in that
way based on the confusion created by the original record. Here is one possibility for revising the original document.

Physical Therapy Note

Date: 1/3/09 _____

Referred by: Dr. _____ with a diagnosis of a Left knee strain _____

Age/Sex: 32/F _____

Precautions:

Insurance: Workers' Compensation

Visit Note: RE-EVALUATION

> **S:** The patient states "my knee still hurts, especially on the outside and I've still got some pain in my low back."
>
> **O:** Patellar mobility and stretching of hip flexors and hamstring.
>
> **A:** Following session, the elevated Left iliac crest was corrected. The patient will see Dr. , on Monday. And to Occupational Health for follow-up later next week.
>
> The patient still has tenderness on her Right tiobio-fibular area, but no tenderness on her inferior patellar bursa. She has a range of motion in the Left knee that is within functional limits. Manual muscle testing shows her hip flexors = 4/4 and knee extensors = 4/4.
>
> **P:** In 4 weeks the staging goals include: (1) Increased strength in Left lower extremity; (2) Independent home exercise program; (3) Continue point of care 1–2 times per week for lower extremity strengthening; (4) We will also continue therapy for core and stabilization exercises.
>
> PLEASE SIGN BELOW IF AGREEABLE TO PLAN OF CARE AND RETURN BY FAX. THANK YOU VERY MUCH
>
> X _____   DR. _____
>
> X _____   _____ , PT.

Skills Application

1. How does your revised note and the alternate above compare to the original in terms of legibility? Why?

   _____

   _____

   _____

   _____

   _____

2. How would you assess the differences for the expected primary and secondary readers between your revision, this alternate, and the original? Why?

_____

_____

_____

_____

_____

3. Do you think eliminating the abbreviations and using a narrative format in the alternate made a difference in terms of communication effectiveness versus the original? If so, how and why? If no, why not?

_____

_____

_____

_____

4. Compare your assessment of the provider–author's professionalism and credibility in the original versus your revision and/or the alternate record above? What specific details are impacting your assessment and why?

_____

_____

_____

_____

5. Do you feel that the original note was complete and accurate (based on the discussion in Chapter 7)? Why, or why not?

_____

_____

_____

_____

This chapter has explored several diverse patient records and sought to help you better understand the value of the authoring process to the end product—the patient record—but also to allow you to recognize the importance of the issues discussed in Chapter 7 and how you can improve your documents and decrease your legal risks. As you no doubt observed in the original note above, using abbreviations that are not common to all primary readers can obfuscate the message and create perception problems for the provider–author. When an audience perceives that an author is trying to confuse the reader or does not care if the reader can interpret the document, then the audience is likely to find the author much less credible as a source of information and call into question his or her professionalism and clinical skills. As we have discussed throughout this text, a patient record is not a static document, but instead it is a dynamic source of information about the patient, the relationship between the provider and the patient, the provider's critical thinking and decision making, and the provider's professional skills and credibility. If you want to help your patients and minimize your legal risks, take the time to practice the authoring process, to review and proofread your documents, and to strive to be as complete and legible in your communication as possible.

Chapter 11

Final Thoughts on the Authoring Process

Be the Audience

This book was intended to help healthcare providers enhance their patient documentation. Regardless of the format (handwritten, dictated and transcribed, or electronic), medical records are intended to inform readers at a minimum about the following:

- A patient's health
- The provider's critical thinking and decision making
- Treatment outcomes or next steps
- Any unexpected or unusual outcomes

This need to effectively communicate with readers requires providers–authors to clearly recognize the intended and expected audiences for each patient document that they create. As discussed in Chapter 2 and throughout this text, the audiences for patient records are not static but instead dynamic and variable based on the patient's wellness or illness, treatment decisions, outcomes, and a multitude of variables.

However, some fundamental understandings about audiences for patient records can be enumerated as starting points for each document's analysis. In general, primary audiences for most patient records can be expected to include the following:

- The provider–author
- Other healthcare providers
- Provider–author's organization's billing personnel
- Health insurance, Medicare, and Medicaid case managers

While secondary audiences for most patient documents are likely to include, at a minimum, the following:

- Supervisors, managers, or quality assurance staff
- Patient and/or family members

- The Joint Commission or government surveyors
- Malpractice attorneys

These multiple readers of patient records, with their diverse expectations, make it imperative for providers–authors to understand their readers' communication needs and to try to meet or exceed them. When providers–authors recognize the importance of creating documents that communicate effectively to the intended audience, the patient records will not only provide necessary information but illustrate the provider–author's credibility, critical thinking, collaboration, and decision making. In addition, patient records that meet or exceed readers' expectations can be expected to enhance the readers' perceptions of the author's professionalism and expertise. And patient records that effectively communicate with the primary and secondary audiences are also likely to lessen the provider–author's malpractice risk. Therefore, the importance of knowing your audiences for each patient record you author is very critical to your role as a healthcare provider. As you know, part of your responsibility, both professionally and legally, is to document what you learned about a patient, what decisions you made and why, and what are the patient's treatment plans and outcomes. This responsibility can best be achieved by understanding and meeting your readers' needs and expectations and by ensuring that your patient documents fulfill their intended purposes and uses.

Each patient record has its own unique purpose and intended use. As discussed in Chapters 2 and 3, it is important for you as the provider–author to analyze the purpose for the document prior to creating it, and to determine how you want it to be used. While the purpose for various patient records will be distinct and based on the type of record being created, the patient's problem, the context, outcomes, and so forth, each document will have specific purposes and uses. Though the purposes may be diverse, the use for almost all patient records will be similar. Specifically, providers–authors will want to ensure that any patient document can be used by readers to

- Gain the expected and needed patient information.
- Understand the provider–author's rationale for decision making, actions–plans.
- Evaluate provider–author's actions and outcomes.
- Illustrate provider–author's credibility and professionalism.
- Decrease malpractice risks.

By carefully analyzing the audience, purpose(s), and use(s) for each document you author prior to creating it, you will have the best opportunity to effectively communicate with your intended audiences and to meet their expectations and needs. And, as we have illustrated and discussed throughout this text, with practice, such an analysis can be done in a minute or two and can enhance the provider–author's communication, credibility, and professionalism.

Authoring Process

In order to meet the provider–author and his or her audiences' needs, in Chapter 3 and throughout this text, we have discussed the importance of developing and using an authoring process for all your patient documentation. To ensure that you are able to analyze the audience, purpose(s), and use(s) for each document you author, as well as to communicate the necessary information that your audience expects, this text has illustrated the value of using a pre-authoring, authoring, revising, and proofreading process. This authoring process is intended not to increase the time required to create patient records, but instead, to help you document the information needed and expected by readers, to fulfill the intended purposes for each record, and to ensure that the document is used as you want it to be. Remember the authoring process involves the following:

1. Pre-authoring analyses
   a. Audiences
      i. Primary
      ii. Secondary
   b. Purposes
      i. Provide patient and provider-related information.
      ii. Meet professional, institutional, and legal requirements.
      iii. Communicate data needed for reimbursement.
      iv. Minimize provider–author's legal risks.
   c. Uses
      i. Communicate provider's critical thinking, decision making, treatments, outcomes, and next steps.
      ii. Aid other healthcare providers in caring for the patient.
      iii. Illustrate provider–author's professional skills and acumen.
      iv. Enhance provider–author's credibility.
      v. Maximize reimbursement for institution and/or provider–author.
      vi. Minimize provider–author's malpractice risks.
   d. Content
      i. Determine what information from a patient needs to be communicated.
      ii. Ensure provider–author's assessments, critical thinking, and plans are clearly documented.
      iii. Evaluate if any unusual circumstances, findings, or events need to be explained and communicated.
2. Authoring
   a. Create a patient record that supplies the expected content for the intended audiences, purposes, and uses.

3. Revising or re-authoring
   a. Whenever possible, review what you authored and revise as needed to achieve your pre-authoring analyses.
4. Proofreading
   a. Ensure that there are
      i. No misspelled words.
      ii. No typos ("their" instead of "there").
      iii. No missing words.
      iv. No unclear abbreviations.
      v. No illegible words or phrases.
      vi. No incomplete or inaccurate statements.
      vii. No erasures or obliterated words or phrases.

The advantages of using an authoring process are many, but specifically, this process can help you assure that you understand

- Who your expected readers for each document will be.
- What are the audiences' expectations and needs.
- What are the most critical purposes for the document.
- How you want your audiences to use the document.
- What information is necessary to communicate for your readers to reach the same conclusions and decisions as you did.
- How to create a patient record that enhances your credibility and minimizes your malpractice risks.

In addition, developing and maintaining an authoring process will prove invaluable regardless of the format for the patient records that you are creating. This process will help enhance your communication effectiveness no matter if you are authoring a handwritten, dictated and transcribed, or electronic patient record. The authoring process can assist you in all aspects of your patient documentation; however, you have to be willing to practice it and utilize it in order to fully benefit from all it has to offer.

Reporter's Formula

One way to help you analyze what information you need to record in your patient documents is to use the Reporter's Formula. This formula seeks answers to some basic questions, and you can determine, based on your patient, the context, circumstances, and so forth, which questions to supply answers for and how much detail you need to describe in order to effectively communicate needed information to your readers. Specifically, the Reporter's Formula seeks answers to the following six questions:

1. What?
2. Where?
3. Why?
4. When?
5. Who?
6. How?

Therefore, you might want to use this formula to remind yourself to communicate the following to your readers:

1. What happened to the patient or what procedure you performed.
2. Where the event happened, or where the injury is on the body, or where your treatment was focused.
3. Why the patient was doing something, or why you made a treatment decision.
4. When the patient first noticed the problem, or when your baseline studies were performed.
5. Who was involved in the incident or accident, or who you referred the patient to.
6. How the accident occurred, how long the symptoms have existed, or how your treatment will be assessed.

These six questions can serve as easy reminders to help you assess what information to include, how much information, and what elements are unnecessary based on the patient's condition, care, or outcome.

Electronic Patient Records

When documenting via an electronic (computerized) patient record, the authoring process can be of great assistance; however, as discussed in Chapter 6, electronic patient records can create their own problems for providers–authors. Too often, authors of these electronic documents are not expert typists, or they have checklist choices that do not meet their record-keeping needs. In such situations, providers–authors should be especially diligent in their proofreading and in trying to find a way to document in a narrative format any additional information that will be important for readers and/or the provider–author in caring for the patient.

While electronic patient records have great potential for enhancing communication legibility, provider–authors need to recognize the current shortcomings associated with electronic documentation:

1. There is no nationwide standard nationwide for electronic record-keeping software.
2. Therefore, most electronic records must be printed for use outside the institution where they were created.

3. Electronic-record software frequently does not include a spell checker.
4. Prior electronic records may not be printed and sent to outside treaters–institutions with the printout of the current record, so current documents need to avoid referring readers to prior documents (and instead include the earlier documentation in the current record).
5. Checklists and other record-keeping options may not offer providers adequate opportunities to fully document the patient's history, physical findings, critical thinking, and so forth.
6. Software programs may not provide options for documenting unusual findings, circumstances, or events.

These potential problems require providers to carefully assess their electronic records and to ensure that the format does not detract from the author's pre-writing analysis, information sharing, and communication goals. Wherever necessary, providers–authors should find a mechanism in the electronic record or otherwise to document the information that he or she feel needs to be in the patient record to communicate effectively with readers.

In addition, the potential ease of use and malpractice risks associated with patient-related e-mail communication, as well as the development of professional or personal websites or social networking, needs to be carefully assessed by each provider. As an electronic documentation of interactions between providers and patients, or providers and consultants about patients, these seemingly simple communication vehicles are associated with possible confidentiality, record keeping, and malpractice risks, and should be discussed with a provider's risk manager or personal attorney prior to implementation.

Legal Considerations

As discussed in Chapter 7, patient records are intended to serve as memory devices for their providers–authors. It may be difficult, years after the event, to recall the specific details about a patient's interview, exam, treatment, and outcome; however, an effectively authored patient record will provide authors with more objective documented information. However, the benefits of a thoroughly authored patient encounter can only be obtained if the provider creates a patient record that details his or her interaction, physical exam findings, critical thinking, and so forth.

In addition to the documentation for later recall, the patient record needs to be authored in a timely manner (as soon after the interaction as possible) and needs to include the specific date and time of the provider–patient interaction, as well as the author's signature and professional title. Similarly, late entries need to be documented as above but must follow your institution's policies and procedures for late entries into the patient record. And, you should similarly assess if the late entry will appear to readers as self-serving, rather than informational.

Furthermore, Chapter 7 describes the importance of complete and accurate record keeping. Readers expect healthcare professionals to document accurately and completely the what, where, why, when, who, and how of each patient encounter. Provider–authors should recognize the perception issues related to incomplete and/or inaccurate record keeping and avoid it. Audiences are likely to question a provider's credibility and professional abilities if she or he cannot completely and accurately document what occurred and why.

Providers–authors need to ensure that their patient records are legible and avoid any confusing or unclear abbreviations. In addition, handwritten records must be legible in order to be useful to intended readers. And authors should avoid erasures and obliterations, which may appear to readers as an attempt to obfuscate the record or to cover up a mistake.

These simple rules can assist you as a patient–author to minimize your malpractice risks. Providers will benefit from patient records that are timely, legible, accurate, and complete. The more you can ensure that your records meet these standards for documentation, the better your chances are at reducing your legal risks.

This book was created to assist you in improving your patient record communication effectiveness. One of the goals of this text was to provide you with a format that you could return to from time to time to practice your patient record-keeping skills. You might want to use this book after you have interviewed and/or examined a patient to help you enhance your documentation of that encounter and to assist you in analyzing your communication about the patient and your findings, critical thinking, decision making, and treatment. Or, you might want to refer to this text if you have an unusual or unexpected event or outcome that you need to document. Finally, the authors wish you much success with your patient records and hope that you find this text beneficial as you strive to develop and/or enhance your document communication effectiveness.

Index